Oakes'

# Neonatal
# Pediatric
*Respiratory Care*

### 7th Edition

Dana Oakes
Scot Jones

RespiratoryBooks.com
*a division of:*
Health Educator Publications, Inc.
476 Shotwell Road
Suite 102, PMB 161
Clayton, NC 27520

P9-CMM-409

# Authors

## Dana F. Oakes, BA, RRT-NPS
*Educational Consultant*

*Formerly:*

**Director of Clinical Education**
Respiratory Care Program
Columbia Union College
Tacoma Park, Maryland

**Educational Coordinator/Instructor**
Respiratory Care Department
Children's Hospital Nat. Medical Center
Washington, D.C.

**Director of Respiratory Care**
VA Medical Center
Washington, D.C.


## Scot N. Jones BA, RRT-ACCS
*Educational Consultant*

*Formerly:*

**Director of Clinical Education**
Respiratory Care Program
Broward College
Coconut Creek, Florida

**Respiratory Care Supervisor**
Respiratory Care Department
Vidant Medical Center
Greenville, NC

---

## ISBN 978-0-932887-54-2

RespiratoryBooks.com
A Division of Health Educator Publications, Inc.
476 Shotwell Drive, PMB 161
Clayton, NC 27520

# Table of Contents
(detailed table of contents at start of each chapter)

## Authors' Acknowledgement

Always first and foremost, we are thankful for our Lord, Jesus Christ, for His allowing us to play this small part in our field, for guiding our hands for over 30 years, and for the tens of thousands that have used this pocket guide clinically. **To Him, and to Him only goes the Glory.**

Dana Oakes and Scot Jones

## Special Dedication

I dedicate this book to the memory of **Leann Gore, RRT**, whose untimely passing was a terrible loss to all of us at Arkansas Children's Hospital, and especially to the babies in the NICU. Her calm demeanor, wonderful sense of humor, and nearly magical ability to troubleshoot the ventilator inspired everyone. We will miss her intensely.

Sherry E. Courtney, MD

## Important Disclaimer:

## Editors

**Sherry E. Courtney, MD**
*Professor of Pediatrics*
*Director, Clinical Research in Neonatology*
Department of Pediatrics
Section of Neonatology
Arkansas Children's Hospital/
University of Arkansas for Medical Sciences

**Rakesh Patel, MD, MBA, RRT**
*Respiratory Therapist*
Memorial Hermann Hospital

## Past Senior Editor

**Jay P. Goldsmith, MD**
*Professor of Pediatrics*
Tulane University

*Chairman*
Department of Pediatrics
Ochsner Clinic

*Co-Director of Nurseries*
Ochsner Foundation Hospital
Case Western Reserve University
Cleveland, Ohio

## Assistant Editors

**Arif Ali, RRT**
*Respiratory Care Practitioner*
*ECMO Specialist*
Joe Dimaggio Children's Hospital
Hollywood, Florida

**Hajar AlTamimi**
*Respiratory Therapy Student (2017)*
University of Hartford,
Hartford, Connecticut

**Amanda Beachner, BS, RRT**
*Respiratory Care Practitioner*
Johnson City Medical Center
Johnson City, Tennessee

**Brittne Berry, BS, RRT**
*Respiratory Care Practitioner*
Children's Healthcare of Atlanta
Atlanta, Georgia

**Edmund Borza, BA, RRT-NPS, ACCS, CPFT**
*Assistant Professor*
Kapi'olani Community College
Honolulu, Hawaii

**Darian Brewington, BS, RRT-NPS**
*Respiratory Care Practitioner (Advanced)*
Vidant Medical Center
Greenville, North Carolina

**Kelsey Campagnola, BS, RRT**
*Respiratory Care Practitioner*
Littleton Adventist Hospital
Littleton, Colorado

**Edwin L. Coombs, Jr., MA, RRT-NPS, ACCS, FAARC**
*Director of Marketing—Intensive Care*
Draeger, Inc.
Telford, Pennsylvania

**Angella T. Crane, BA, RRT-NPS**
*NICU Respiratory Therapist*
Community North Hospital
Indianapolis, Indiana

**Frank DiLorenzo, RRT-NPS, C-NPT**
*Neonatal/Pediatric Transport Supervisor*
Florida Hospital for Children
Orlando, Florida

**Joseph Enzweig, RRT, RCP**
*Instructor*
Respiratory Therapy Program
St. Philip's College
San Antonio, Texas

**Dana Evans, MHA, RRT-NPS**
*Respiratory Care Director*
Ann & Robert H. Lurie Children's Hospital
Chicago, Illinois

**Angelic Feliciano, RRT**
*Respiratory Care Practitioner*
Johns Hopkins All Children's Hospital
St. Petersburg, Florida

**Kimberly S. Firestone, MSc, RRT**
*Neonatal Respiratory Outreach Clinical Liaison*
Akron Children's Hospital
Akron, Ohio

**Tashina Gentry, BS, RRT**
*Respiratory Care Practitioner*
Arkansas Children's Hospital
Little Rock, Arkansas

**Shivani Hira, BS, RRT**
*Respiratory Care Practitioner*
Dell Children's Medical Center
St. David's Children's North Austin Med Center
Austin, Texas

**Robb Johnson, BS, CCP, RRT**
*Staff Perfusionist*
New York Presbyterian Columbia University Medical Center
New York City, New York

**Simon Kozee, RRT-NPS**
*Ventilator Sales Executive*
Draeger, Inc.
Telford, Pennsylvania

**Rhianna R. Lees, RRT-NPS**
*Respiratory Care Practitioner*
Newark Beth Israel Medical Center and Children's Hospital
Newark, New Jersey

**Yanyun Lin, BS, RRT, RPSGT**
*Sleep Technologist*
White Plains Hospital
White Plains, New York

**Maggie Minnette, RRT**
*Respiratory Care Practitioner*
Deaconess Hospital
Evansville, Indiana

**Stephanie B. Moore, RRT-NPS**
*Respiratory Care Practitioner*
*ECMO Specialist*
Vidant Medical Center
Greenville, North Carolina

**Karly Murphy**
*Respiratory Care Practitioner*
Alberta Health Services
Edmonton, Alberta

**Sara Wing Parker, MPH, RRT-NPS, AE-C**
*Assistant Clinical Professor*
University of Missouri
Columbia, Missouri

**Lee Anne Pate, MEd, RRT**
*Assistant Professor*
*Director of Clinical Education*
Respiratory Therapy Program
Shawnee State University
Portsmouth, Ohio

**Mega Patel, BS, RRT**
*Respiratory Care Practitioner*
Mount Carmel Health Systems
Columbus, Ohio

**Swara Patel, BS, RRT**
*Respiratory Care Practitioner*
Bergen Regional Medical Center
Paramus, New Jersey

**Kellee J Rickerly, BA, RRT**
*Director of Clinical Education*
Lane Community College
Respiratory Therapy Program
Eugene, Oregon

**John Rutkowski, MBA, MPA, RRT, CPFT, FACHE, FAARC**
*Assistant Chair Allied Health*
*Respiratory Therapy Program Director*
County College of Morris
Randoph, New Jersey

**John Salyer, MBA, RRT-NPS, FAARC**
*Senior Clinical Analyst*
*Formerly: Respiratory Therapy Director*
Seattle Children's Hospital and Research Institute
Seattle, Washington

**Sean Shortall, RRT-NPS, RPFT**
*Respiratory Care Practitioner*
St. Joseph's Hospital
Bangor, Maine

**Baylie E. Sosa, RRT, RCP**
*Respiratory Care Practitioner*
Corona Regional Hospital
Corona, California

**Howard Stein, MD**
*Director of Neonatology and Neonatal Transport*
ProMedica Toledo Children's Hospital
Toledo, Ohio

**Matt Steringa**
*Sleep Clinician*
Provincial Sleep Group
Edmonton, Alberta

**Marcus Stowe, MS, RRT-NPS, ACCS**
*Associate Professor*
Respiratory Care Program
School of Health Sciences
Ivy Tech Community College
Lawrence, Indiana

**Ambyr Tolleson, RRT**
*Respiratory Care Practitioner*
Florida Hospital for Children
Orlando, Florida

**Chris Webb, RRT, RCP**
*Respiratory Care Practitioner*
Pomona Valley Hospital
Pomona, California

**Brie Webster, BS, RRT**
*Respiratory Care Practitioner*
Banner Thunderbird Medical Center
Glendale, Arizonaa

# 1 Neonatal Resuscitation

CONTENTS

Neonatal

Resuscitation

**Notes:**

## Neonatal Resuscitation Algorithm
*Adapted from 2016 AHA Guidelines*

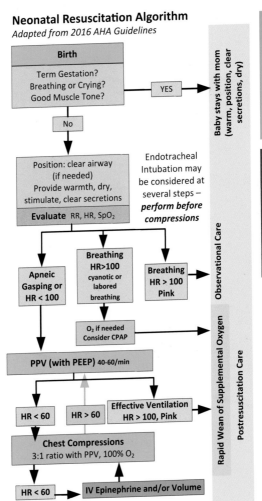

**Birth**

Term Gestation?
Breathing or Crying?
Good Muscle Tone?

YES → Baby stays with mom (warm, position, clear secretions, dry)

No

Position: clear airway (if needed)
Provide warmth, dry, stimulate, clear secretions
**Evaluate** RR, HR, SpO₂

Endotracheal Intubation may be considered at several steps – *perform before compressions*

**Apneic Gasping or HR < 100**

**Breathing HR>100** cyanotic or labored breathing

**Breathing HR > 100 Pink**

O₂ if needed Consider CPAP

**PPV (with PEEP)** 40-60/min

HR < 60

HR > 60

**Effective Ventilation HR > 100, Pink**

**Chest Compressions** 3:1 ratio with PPV, 100% O₂

HR < 60

**IV Epinephrine and/or Volume**

Neonatal

Resuscitation

Observational Care

Rapid Wean of Supplemental Oxygen

Postresuscitation Care

## Targeted Preductal SpO$_2$ after Birth

Oxygen administration should be guided by SpO$_2$ (pulse oximeter on upper right extremity—such as wrist or palm)

| Time | Target SpO$_2$ |
|------|------|
| 1 minute | 60-65% |
| 2 minutes | 65-70% |
| 3 minutes | 70-75% |
| 4 minutes | 75-80% |
| 5 minutes | 80-85% |
| 10 minutes | 85-95% |

**Summary of Neonatal Resuscitation Guidelines[1]:**
1. **Preparation and Team Briefing**
2. **Initial Steps**
3. **Use of Positive-Pressure Ventilation (PPV)**
4. **Chest Compressions**
5. **Drugs Administered**
6. **Post-Resuscitation Care**
7. **Ethics / Discontinuation**

## 1. Preparation and Team Briefing

- Verify that all supplies are available and that equipment is functional
- Every birth should be attended by at least one person who can perform resuscitation
- Every high-risk birth should be attended by a team of people who can perform resuscitation, with a team leader identified, and a briefing performed

## 2. Initial Steps

> **Body temperature goal:** 36.5 - 37.5° C
> **Dry/Stimulate**
> **Avoid routine suctioning**
> **Careful oxygen administration**

- Neonatal body temperature should be maintained between 36.5 C- 37.5 C with no asphyxia, particularly in neonates < 32 wks gestation. Radiant warmers, plastic wrap, thermal mattresses, warmed humidified gases are all reasonable strategies. NOTE that hyperthermia is a risk.
- <u>Routine</u> suctioning (bulb syringe or catheter) is not recommended, regardless of presence of meconium-stained amniotic fluid. Greatest emphasis is on initiating ventilation within 1st minute of life.
- Heart rate can best be monitored using a 3-lead ECG, while oxygenation can be best monitored using pulse oximetry. Increase in HR is seen as a very sensitive measure of success in resuscitation efforts.

---

[1] These are summarized from the American Heart Association Neonatal Resuscitation Program, published November, 2015.

- Oxygen administration should be maintained within a safe range (no hypoxia, no hyperoxia). Use targeted ranges on page 1-4.
  - ≥ 35 wks: Start with Room Air (RA)
  - < 35 wks: Start with 21-30%
  - If $SpO_2$ is not in target range, start with 30% (free-flow @ 10 L/min). If $SpO_2$ is still below range and on 100%, trial CPAP. If baby is not breathing, use PPV (below).

## 3. Use of Positive Pressure Ventilation (PPV)

**Manually ventilate** 40-60 breaths/min
**Use CPAP/PEEP** with pre-term neonates

### Manual Resuscitation

- Rates of 40-60 breaths/min are most common
- Increase of HR > 100/min is best indicator of success
- Use enough pressure to see gentle rise of chest
- Start with 5-6 cmH$_2$O PEEP in preterm neonates
- Auscultate HR (over heart) for 1st 15 seconds—check for an increasing HR
- Understand how to properly use the type of resuscitator available in the delivery room
- If < 30 weeks consider having surfactant ready

### Intubation

- Consider intubating when unable to ventilate effectively, or no improvement with bag-valve-mask, when compressions are performed, and in unique situations (congenital diaphragmatic hernia, for example)
- Exhaled $CO_2$ is the recommended method of confirming ET Tube placement (except if perfusion is poor, such as during cardiac arrest). Other methods include chest movement, breath sounds, and condensate in ET tube.
- Remember, the vocal cord indicator on an ET Tube is an estimation of placement and should not be used to confirm placement

## 4. Chest Compressions

> **Technique:** 2-thumb technique preferred
> **Depth:** ⅓ A-P diameter on lower 3rd of sternum
> **Rate:** 120 combined compressions + breaths per minute
> **Synchronize with compressions** (3:1 ratio)

- Compressions are indicated when HR < 60/min despite adequate ventilation
- 100% $O_2$ is indicated during compressions (wean aggressively once HR recovers)
- Compressions should be delivered on lower third of sternum, with a depth of ~⅓ A-P diameter
- 2-thumb technique is preferred method (do not use 2-finger technique)
- Coordinate compressions/ventilations at a ratio of 3:1 (120 events per minute) unless cardiac in origin (then use 15:2)
- RR, HR, $SpO_2$ should be reassessed periodically, but avoid frequent interruptions

## 5. Drugs Administered

- Drug administration is uncommon as bradycardia is usually caused by ventilation issues/hypoxemia
- The use of epinephrine and/or volume is indicated when HR < 60/min despite ventilation with 100% $O_2$ and chest compressions

## SEE DRUGS NEXT PAGE

## Epinephrine
*Epinephrine is considered after PPV and compressions have been trialed (see NRP algorithm).*

1:10 000 Epinephrine by IV:
 **0.1 - 0.3 mL/kg**

1:10 000 Epinephrine by ET Tube:
 **0.3 - 1 mL/kg**

**1:10 000 Epinephrine = 0.1 mg/mL**

## Volume Expansion
*Volume expansion is considered when blood loss is known or suspected, and heart rate has not responded otherwise. Early administration increases risk of intraventricular hemorrhage.*

Isotonic Crystalloid Solution   or
Blood

**10 mL/kg**/dose

## 6. Post-Resuscitation Care
- IV glucose infusion should be considered to avoid hypoglycemia (which increases risk of brain injury)
- Therapeutic hypothermia should be considered with moderate-to-severe hypoxic-ischemic encephalopathy

## 7. Ethics / Discontinuation
- If it is believed there is no chance for survival, resuscitation should not be offered
- If there is a questionable risk for survival, parents should be included in the decision-making process regarding resuscitation efforts

## CONTENTS

## ■ Summary of Lung Development

Lungs are filled with fluid until first breath at birth
(250-300 mL is secreted/day)

| Stage | Estimated Time Period | Major Events |
|-------|----------------------|--------------|
| Embryonal | 3-7 wks | Trachea and Bronchi form |
| Pseudo-glandular | 7-17 wks | Further branching / terminal bronchioles form<br><br>NO respiratory bronchioles or alveoli yet |
| Canalicular | 17-26 wks | Respiratory bronchioles form, which divide into alveolar ducts<br><br>Some surfactant (Type II cells) form around 22 wks |
| Saccular | 26-40 wks | Terminal sacs (roughly alveoli) form, capillaries bond to alveolar sacs<br><br>Surfactant production increases |
| Alveolar | 33 wks - until about 8-years-old | Alveoli develop. Full maturity doesn't occur until about 8-years-old. |

# ■ Neonatal Age Determination

## Gestational Age

From date of conception (see below for ways to calculate this) This is usually an estimation.

| Age of viability[1] | 22-23 weeks |
|---|---|
| Preterm[2] | < 37 weeks |
| Term | 37-42 weeks |
| Postterm | > 42 weeks |

[1]Note there is debate about whether to resuscitate these infants. Neonates born at < 22 weeks have a zero or near-zero chance of survival.
[2]Some studies suggest designating 34 0/7 weeks to 36 6/7 weeks as "Late Preterm" with an emphasis on careful monitoring (Engle, 2016)

**Important Note:** Gestational age is often presented as WEEKS and DAYS. There is no consensus on the presentation, so may be presented as:

- 34 weeks, 5 days
- 34 5/7
- 34 +5
- 34.5 (the # days is after decimal point, not a decimal %)

## Determining Estimated Gestational Age (EGA)

Most common methods:

### From Last Menstrual Period (PMA, post-menstrual age)
- Traditional method
- Tends to over-estimate actual gestational age

### From Ultrasound
- More accurate method
- Uses anatomic measurements (biparietal diameter and head circumference) and physiologic activity (presence of heart-beat, for example)

## By Weight

| | |
|---|---|
| Very Low Birth Weight (VLBW): | < 1500 g |
| Extremely Low Birth Weight (ELBW): | < 800 g |

## Corrected Age

Some clinicians use "corrected age" (adjusted) which corrects for prematurity

**Actual Age in Weeks  -  Weeks of Prematurity = Corrected Age**

| student tip | developmental milestones |
|---|---|

It is important to understand the age you are using.  A neonate born at 26-weeks but is now 4 months old is not at the same developmental milestones as a 4-month old born full-term (for example, eating baby food).  However, this does not mean that the baby is lagging behind developmentally.

# ■ General Anticipated Issues by Gestational Age*

| Gestational Age (wks) | 23 | 24 | 25 | 26 | 27 | 28 | 29+ |
|---|---|---|---|---|---|---|---|
| **Respiratory** | | | | | | | |
| **Lack of Surfactant** *surfactant is detectable at ~24 wks, but does not reach a fully functional level until ~35 wks* | | | | | | | |
| **Apnea (of Prematurity)** *may be present until 43 wks gestation - usually more severe with extreme prematurity* | | | | | | | |
| **Need for Vent Support** *initiation of some type of PPV: N-CPAP or invasive ventilation* | | | | | | | |
| **Cardiac** | | | | | | | |
| **PDA/murmur** *may or may not require intervention* | | | | | | | |
| **Hypotension** *especially hypotension requiring pressors* | | | | | | | |
| **Neurological** | | | | | | | |
| Head Bleed | | | | | | | |
| **Other** | | | | | | | |
| Thermoregulation | | | | | | | |

*Very general guidelines based on review of relevant studies/data. There are many factors that need to be considered, including the baby's size/weight, method of delivery, etc.

Red = > 75% incidence in gestational age group
Orange = around 50% incidence in gestational age group
Yellow = around 25-30% incidence in gestational age group
Green = < 25% incidence in gestational age group

Neonatal

Assessment

# ■ Fetal Heart Rate Monitoring

Fetal Heart Rate (FHR) is monitored during labor and is of particular importance in high risk situations. There are two primary ways to monitor the fetal heart rate:

1. Externally: Sensors are strapped to the mother's abdomen. These use doppler technology (sound) or a fetoscope (similar to a stethoscope). Accuracy depends on a number of factors, including movement.

2. Internally: Sensor is attached directly to the fetal skin (usually scalp). This direct method is usually more accurate. Note that it requires rupture of the membranes and is invasive.

FHR monitoring is done with contractions to determine variability.

**Monitor and Assess:**
  A. Baseline Fetal Heart Rate
  B. Baseline Variability
  C. Periodic Changes

**A. Baseline Fetal Heart Rate**: This is the FHR in the absence of uterine contractions (and between any periodic rate changes)

|  | Rate (bpm) | With Decelerations* | |
|---|---|---|---|
|  |  | Yes | No |
| **Tachycardia** | > 160 | Ominous** Give $O_2$ | Usually Benign *Monitor Pt* |
| **Normal Baseline** | 120-160 |  |  |
| **Bradycardia** | < 120 | Ominous** Give $O_2$ | Usually Benign *Monitor* |

*Decelerations refer to a drop in the FHR <u>when</u> the deceleration occurs is an important consideration during the assessment.

**Tachycardia or Bradycardia with decelerations suggest possible fetal asphyxia:
<u>Maternal causes</u>: anemia, anesthesia, hemorrhage, hypertension, hypotension, hyperthermia, supine position
<u>Fetal causes</u>: cord or head compression, placental separation, post-maturity

**B. Baseline Variability**: This is the variation of the FHR from one beat to the next. It is an indicator of the health of the fetus at any particular moment. **Variability is a healthy sign.**

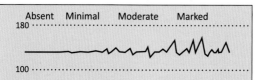

| Variability | Average rate variability between beats (bpm) | Common Causes  *Interventions* |
|---|---|---|
| **Absent** | undetectable | Severe fetal distress **Ominous**  *Consider immediate delivery* |
| **Minimal** | < 5 (detectable) | Fetal sleep cycle Drugs (analgesics, atropine, barbiturates, narcotics, tranquilizers)  *Monitor closely Discontinue drugs Stimulate Fetus Change Mom's position* |
| **Moderate (normal)** | 6-25 | |
| **Marked** | > 25 | Fetal stimulation (activity)  *No intervention needed* |

### Representative FHR tracing showing variability

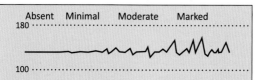

**C. Periodic Changes in FHR:** Changes usually related to uterine contractions (normally there is no relationship). See illustration next page.

|  | Causes | Significance *(Interventions)* |
|---|---|---|
| **Acceleration** | Fetal movement | Indicates well-being |
|  | Abdominal palpation or vaginal exam | Benign |
|  | Partial umbilical vein compression (such as breech) | Usually benign but may become more severe *(observe closely)* |
| **Deceleration Early** | Compression of head against cervix | Benign |
| **Deceleration Late** | ↓ placental perfusion: compression, maternal position, oxytocin, post-mature Maternal diabetes, anemia, hypertension, hypotension Placenta previa Placental abruption | Ominous *(Administer O₂, obtain fetal ABG, Change maternal position [elevate legs]]) Consider early delivery if persistent* |
| **Deceleration Variable** | **Compression of umbilical cord:** | |
|  | FHR > 80 bpm for < 30 sec | Mild: common and benign |
|  | FHR 60-80 bpm for 30-60 sec | Moderate *(Change mom's position)* |
|  | FHR < 60 bpm for > 60 sec | Repetitive Moderate or Severe: *(Administer O₂ to mom, get fetal ABG, Immediate delivery? )* |

## FHR Deceleration Types

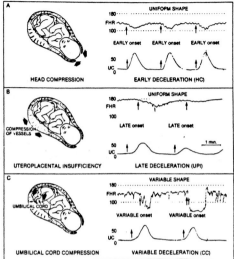

Reprinted with permission. Hon, E. An Atlas of Fetal Heart Rate Patterns.
© 1968 Horty Press.

### Explanations:

- The **top** tracing for each of the above is Fetal Heart Rate (marked FHR). The numbers (100-180) represent the HR in beats per minute.
- The **bottom** tracing for each of the above is Uterine Contractions (marked UC). The numbers (0-50) represent mm Hg—a measure of pressure. These are reflective of the strength and number of contractions.

## Summary of Fetal Monitoring

| Pattern | Indicators |
|---------|-----------|
| **Reassuring** | FHR baseline normal (120-160 bpm)<br>Average baseline variability<br>Early decelerations only -or-<br>    Mild variable decelerations -or-<br>    Accelerations<br>Fetal pH 7.25-7.30 |
| **Non-Reassuring** | FHR baseline outside normal<br>Progressive ↓ in baseline variability<br>Fetal pH 7.15-7.25 |
| **Ominous** | Severe bradycardia<br>Prolonged deceleration -or-<br>    Severe variable deceleration -or-<br>    Late deceleration<br>Fetal pH < 7.15 |

## STUDENT tip

Most of the time we use grams when talking about neonates under 1 kg. Converting is easy: 1 kg = 1000 grams. Move the decimal point 3 spots to the right and you have grams.

**Grams to Kilograms:** Move decimal point 3 places to the left

Example:
A 34 week neonate is born weighing 0.5 kg. This is equivalent to 500 grams.

## ■ Fetal Lung Maturity (Summary of Tests)

*note that the clinical value of determining lung maturity is directly related to the risk of developing Respiratory Distress Syndrome (RDS)*

| Test | Result (normal pregnancy) | Comments |
|------|--------------------------|----------|
| **Lamellar Body Count**<br><br>***MOST COMMON TEST*** | > 50,000 mcL indicates maturity | Surfactant is packaged into lamellar bodies. The presence of lamellar bodies in amniotic fluid correlates to the presence of surfactant<br><br>Consider use of L/S ratio if results are inconclusive (30,000-50,000) |
| **Lecithin/ Sphingomyelin (L/S) Ratio** | S > L until 26 wks<br>S = L until ~36 wks<br>L > S by 36 wks | Ratio > 2.0 indicates fetal lung maturity<br><br>False positive when contaminated with maternal/fetal blood or vaginal secretions |
| **Phosphatidyl-glycerol (PG)** | reported + or -<br>OR<br>$\geq 0.5$ indicates maturity | Helpful if complicated by maternal diabetes<br><br>No false ↑ as seen with L/S ratio |
| **Foam Stability Index** | > 0.48 at maturity | This is a measure of the stability of surfactant and ethanol, suggesting maturity<br><br>Do NOT use silicone tubes (false foam forms) |
| **Amniotic Fluid Shake Test** | Complete ring of bubbles at 1:2 dilution | Indicates presence of surfactant, but not amount. Quick, bedside test |

## ■ Stages of Labor and Delivery

**Normal Labor and Delivery**

| Stage | Key Events |
|-------|-----------|
| **Stage I**<br><br>7-18 hrs* | **True Contractions¹:**<br><br>Latent Phase<br>• mild<br>• irregular to start<br>• ~ every 10-15<br>Active Phase<br>• more rhythmic<br>• stronger<br>• ↑ frequency<br><br>**Cervix:**<br>effacement (stretching - measured in %)<br>        (100% effaced is fully stretched)<br>dilation (widening - measured in cm)<br>        (3-4 cm is active; 10 cm is complete) |
| **Stage II**<br><br>20 min-<br>3 hrs* | Contractions increase in strength and frequency<br>Descent of fetus through birth canal<br>    head-down (vertex) position²<br>    face-down once in birth canal<br>    upper shoulders deliver, then lower, then body<br>Umbilical cord is clamped, initiating CV changes |
| **Stage III**<br><br>3-30 min | Contractions continue<br>Delivery of placenta |

\* There are some differences between nulli- and multipara preg.

¹**False contractions:** called Braxton Hicks contractions, also known as prodromal labor, are sporadic uterine contractions

²**Breech position:** baby presents with bottom first (buttocks with feet/legs folded up, or feet/legs first). This position increases risk of umbilical cord prolapse, usually necessitating a Caesarean section delivery

**Abnormal Labor and Delivery (selected)**

| Prematurity | Stopping Labor (tocolysis)<br>    drug therapy (pharmacology)<br>    positioning (bedrest, etc.) |
|---|---|
| Prolonged Delivery<br>Stage I + II > 20 hrs | Fetal presentation (breech, etc.)<br>Fetal size (macrosomia, etc.)<br>Abnormal contractions<br>Pelvis abnormalities (size, shape) |
| Umbilical Cord | Prolapse (common with breech)<br>    compression ($\downarrow O_2$ supply) |
| Placenta | Placenta Previa (covers cervix)<br>Abruptio Placentae (separates)<br>Preeclampsia (secondary to HTN) |

## ■ High-Risk Delivery (Steps)

1. **Assess Risk and Intervene**
   ***See Next Pages***
   Review the risks associated with delivery
   Intevene pharmacologically as appropriate
   Consider transport of mom as appropriate

2. **Prepare the Team Once Delivery is Likely**
   Team members should be appropriately trained
   Team members should be in place prior to delivery
   Team members should be briefed on risks

3. **Prepare the Equipment**
   ***See Page 2-17***
   Confirm or reconfirm equipment is in place and working

4. **Accept Delivery of Baby**
   Focus is on warming, stimulating, and assessing
   See Neonatal Resuscitation (Chapter 1) for NRP algorithm

# 1. Assess Risk and Intervene

## Goals (as clinically appropriate)

| Delay delivery | Allows baby to mature further Maternal Interventions **DO NOT DELAY with fetal distress** |
|---|---|
| **Perform safe delivery with appropriate professionals and equipment ready** | Transfer high-risk mom/baby to a qualified facility (case-by-case, often by how imminent delivery is) |

## Factors that May Indicate High-Risk

### Pre-delivery Conditions[1]:

- High Blood Pressure (increases risk of preeclampsia)
- Diabetes (gestational or other)
- Autoimmune diseases (lupus, MS, HIV)
- Thyroid disease (uncontrolled)
- Maternal age < 19 years or > 35 years
- Consumption of drugs or medications
- Post-term gestation
- Multiple gestation
- Previous fetal/neonatal death
- Polyhydramnios or oligohydramnios
- Premature rupture of membranes (PROM)
- Maternal infection or illness
- Known or suspected fetal malformations
- Noted diminished fetal activity

### Delivery Conditions[1]:

- Labor at < 32 weeks
- Emergent Caesarean section
- Prolonged PROM
- Fetal distress (FHR monitoring)
- Bleeding (significant)
- Placental abruption
- Meconium-stained amniotic fluid
- Umbilical cord prolapse/nuchal cord
- Anticipated low or high birth weight

[1]Adapted from American Academy of Pediatrics

## Agents Used to Address Preterm labor

| Class of Drug | Typical Drugs | Rationale |
|---|---|---|
| Hormone | Progesterone (vaginally) | Prophylactic, high risk patients, helps mature lungs |
| Antenatal Corticosteroids | Dexamethasone Betamethasone | Matures Lung<br><br>*Repeated doses may cause neonate to be smaller but growth catches up over time* |
| Antibiotics | various | Useful with PPROM |
| **Tocolytic Drugs** *(supress premature labor to allow baby to more fully mature)* | | |
| Beta-Adrenergic Agonists | Terbutaline IV | Relaxes smooth muscle |
| Electrolyte | Magnesium Sulfate | Decreases contractility by interfering with calcium<br><br>*Neonates may show signs of magnesium toxicity (respiratory and/or neuromuscular depression)* |
| Calcium Channel Blockers | Nifedipine (unlabeled use) | Relaxes smooth muscle by inhibiting the influx and release of calcium |
| COX Inhibitor | Indomethacin | Relaxes smooth muscle by inhibiting release of calcium |

PPROM = Preterm Premature Rupture of the Membranes

## Gravidity and Parity

There are a number of ways to quickly consider maternal risk factors. These notations are used to provide maternal history, an important indicator of high-risk pregnancy/delivery.

### GPA System

| G | Gravidity | # of total pregnancies |
|---|---|---|
| P | Preterm Births | # Preterm deliveries (viability up through 37 wks) |
| A | Abortions/ Miscarriages | # Surgical abortions AND miscarriages |

### GTPAL*

| G | Gravidity | # of total pregnancies |
|---|---|---|
| T | Term Births | # Full term deliveries (38+ wks) |
| P | Preterm Births | # Preterm deliveries (viability up through 37 wks) |
| A | Abortions/ Miscarriages | # Surgical abortions AND miscarriages |
| L | Living Children | # Living children |

*Some systems use TPAL, leaving off the Gravidity.

*Example: A 35-year-old is giving birth to a 4th child. Her first pregnancy ended in a miscarriage, the second pregnancy resulted in twins at 39 weeks, and the third resulted in the birth of her daughter at 32 weeks.*

*This would be noted as:*
*G4 T2 P1, A1 L3*

## 2. Prepare the Team

the high-risk delivery team should be assembled with adequate advanced notice to ensure preparations

## 3. Prepare the Equipment

**General Equipment/Supplies:**
- Drugs: epinephrine (1:10,000, 3 mL or 10 mL)
- Radiant warmer (pre-heated)
- Receiving blankets (pre-warmed)
- Stethoscope (neonatal)

**Bag and Mask** (checked and ready):
- Neonatal-sized resuscitaiton bag - *pressure limited*
- Several masks (neonatal, newborn)

**Oxygen** (connected and ready):
- Oxygen source
- Oxygen blender (Air:Oxygen)
- Oxygen tubing
- Pulse oximeter with multiple probes

**Suction equipment**
- Bulb syringe
- Catheters (Suction: 5F, 6F, 8F, 10F)
- Meconium aspirator

**Intubation** (checked and ready):
- Laryngoscopes and Miller blades (#00, #0, #1)
- ET Tubes (2.5, 3.0, 3.5, 4.0) - stylet is optional
- $CO_2$ detector
- Laryngeal Mask Airway (1.0, 1.5) with 5 cc syringe
- Lubricant
- Securing device (tape, etc.)

## 4. Accept Delivery of the baby

Follow NRP Algorithm (SEE page 1-3)

# Pounds (Lbs) and Ounces to Grams

| Lbs | \\ Ounces | | | | | | | | | | | | | | | |
|---|---|---|---|---|---|---|---|---|---|---|---|---|---|---|---|---|
|  | 0 | 1 | 2 | 3 | 4 | 5 | 6 | 7 | 8 | 9 | 10 | 11 | 12 | 13 | 14 | 15 |
| 0 | 0 | 28 | 57 | 85 | 113 | 142 | 170 | 198 | 227 | 255 | 284 | 312 | 340 | 369 | 397 | 425 |
| 1 | 454 | 482 | 510 | 539 | 567 | 595 | 624 | 652 | 680 | 709 | 737 | 765 | 794 | 822 | 850 | 879 |
| 2 | 907 | 936 | 964 | 992 | 1021 | 1049 | 1077 | 1106 | 1134 | 1162 | 1191 | 1219 | 1247 | 1276 | 1304 | 1332 |
| 3 | 1361 | 1389 | 1417 | 1446 | 1474 | 1503 | 1531 | 1559 | 1588 | 1616 | 1644 | 1673 | 1701 | 1729 | 1758 | 1786 |
| 4 | 1814 | 1843 | 1871 | 1899 | 1928 | 1956 | 1984 | 2013 | 2041 | 2070 | 2098 | 2126 | 2155 | 2183 | 2211 | 2240 |
| 5 | 2268 | 2296 | 2325 | 2353 | 2381 | 2410 | 2438 | 2466 | 2495 | 2523 | 2551 | 2580 | 2608 | 2637 | 266 | 2693 |
| 6 | 2722 | 2750 | 2778 | 2807 | 2835 | 2863 | 2892 | 2920 | 2949 | 2977 | 3005 | 3034 | 3062 | 3091 | 3119 | 3147 |
| 7 | 3175 | 3203 | 3232 | 3260 | 3289 | 3317 | 3345 | 3374 | 3402 | 3430 | 3459 | 3487 | 3515 | 3544 | 3572 | 3600 |
| 8 | 3629 | 3657 | 3685 | 3714 | 3742 | 3770 | 3799 | 3827 | 3856 | 3884 | 3912 | 3941 | 3969 | 3997 | 4026 | 4054 |
| 9 | 4082 | 4111 | 4139 | 4167 | 4196 | 4224 | 4252 | 4281 | 4309 | 4337 | 4366 | 4394 | 4423 | 4451 | 4479 | 4508 |
| 10 | 4536 | 4564 | 4593 | 4621 | 4649 | 4678 | 4706 | 4734 | 4763 | 4791 | 4819 | 4848 | 4876 | 4904 | 4933 | 4961 |

**Grams to Kilograms:** Move decimal point 3 places to the left

**Pounds to Grams:** Pounds/.0022  If using Ounces, use DECIMAL EQUIVALENT (for example: 3lb, 8oz = 3.5 lbs NOT 3.8 lbs)

1 lb = 16 oz

## ◼ Cardiovascular Changes at Birth

**Action: Umbilical cord is clamped.**

1. **Ductus venosus** closes and becomes a ligament
   Failure: Patent Ductus Venosus
2. **Ductus arteriosus** closes functionally quickly (may take days in premies). Becomes ligament and permanently closes within 2-4 months.
   Failure: Patent Ductus Arteriosis (PDA)
3. **Foramen ovale** closes functionally quickly. Anatomically seals within 3 months.
   Failure: Patent Foramen Ovale (PFO)
4. **Major increase in pulmonary circulation.** Pulmonary arteries dilate to increase flow from 10% to 100% of cardiac output.
5. **Decreased pulmonary circulation.**
   Failure: Persisitent Pulmonary Hypertension of Newborn (PPHN)

Neonatal

Assessment

## ◼ Pulmonary Changes at Birth

**Action: Baby passes through birth canal (vaginal birth)**

1. **Some Fetal lung fluid is expelled** (squeeze by birth canal) *some is drained through lymphatic system*
   C-Section: may require additional interventions if fetal lung fluid is not expelled or absorbed. Highly individualized.

**Action: Baby takes initial breath (vaginal birth or c-section)**

1. **Inflation of lungs** draws blood into thorax (pressure creates a negative vacuum)
2. **Establishment of air/liquid interface** with surfactant, breaths become progressively easier
3. **Active gas exchange** occurs

## ▨ Fetal Shunts

## Summary of 3 Shunts

1. **Ductus Venosus:** blood shunts around liver (instead of through it)

2. **Foramen Ovale:** blood shunts from right atrium to left atrium (instead of into right ventricle, then pulmonary circulation)

3. **Ductus Arteriosis:** blood shunts from pulmonary artery into the aorta (instead of into pulmonary circulation, then left side of heart)

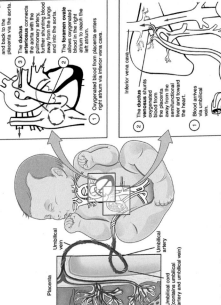

④ Mixed blood travels to the head and body, and back to the placenta via the aorta.

③ The **ductus arteriosus** connects the aorta with the pulmonary artery, further shunting blood away from the lungs and into the aorta.

② The **foramen ovale** allows oxygenated blood in the right atrium to reach the left atrium.

① Oxygenated blood from placenta enters right atrium via inferior vena cava.

Inferior vena cava

② The **ductus venosus** shunts oxygenated blood from the placenta away from the semifunctional liver and toward the heart.

① Blood arrives via umbilical vein.

Umbilical vein

Umbilical artery

Placenta

Umbilical cord (contains umbilical artery and umbilical vein)

*Used under open license from Openstax College, Wikimedia Commons*

2-20

# ◼ Neonatal Anatomy/Physiology (Overview)

| Structure | Characteristic | Clinical Significance |
|-----------|----------------|----------------------|
| Nose | Obligatory nasal breathers | Poor tolerance to obstruction Treatments should be focused on nasal application (unless invasive) |
| Tongue | Relatively large | Neck extension may not effectively relieve obstruction |
| Head | Relatively large | Moving head forward (anterior flexion) may cause airway obstruction |
| Epiglottis | Relatively large & U-shaped | More susceptible to trauma and forms more acute angle with vocal cords |
| Larynx | More anterior and cephalad | Intubation more difficult |
| Cricoid | Narrowest portion of airway | ↑ Resistance with airway edema or infection. Acts as "cuff" during tracheal intubation. |
| Trachea | Small diameter (6 mm) High compliance | ↑ Resistance with airway edema or infection. Collapses easily with neck hyperflexion or hyperextension. |
| Alveoli | ↑ Closing capacity No pores of Kohn | ↑ Air trapping and ↓ collateral circulation of air |
| Pulmonary vessels | ↑ PVR | Very sensitive to constriction by hypoxia, acidosis & hypercarbia |

| Structure | Characteristic | Clinical Significance |
|-----------|----------------|----------------------|
| Chest wall | ↑ Compliance due to weak rib cage<br><br>↑ A-P diameter<br>Ribs horizontal | Breathing is all diaphramatic (abdominal). FRC determined solely by elastic recoil of lungs. Chest wall collapses with neg. pressures. |
| Work of breathing | Increases at lower rates. Weak respiratory muscles | ↑ RR equals early sign of respiratory distress |
| Regulation of breathing | Response to ↓$O_2$ is minimal<br><br>Response to ↑$CO_2$ is minimal in premie | Tolerates hypoxia poorly<br>Apneic spells |

## Assessment

### ▮ APGAR scoring

*This section is summarized from Watterberg KL, Aucott S, Benitz WE, Cummings JJ, Eichenwald EC, Goldsmith J, et al. The Apgar Score. Pediatrics 2015;134(4):819-822*

> **Intervention should not wait for the assignment of an APGAR score.**

- APGAR scores are generally done at 1 min and 5 mins after birth. If < 7 at 5 mins, repeat every 5 minutes for up to 20 minutes.
- Note that an APGAR during resuscitation may index the response to resuscitation, but has otherwise limited use during resuscitation (it is not accurate)
- The APGAR is not intended to be predictive of future disability

# APGAR Scoring (further explanations on previous page)

| Sign | Score | | |
|---|---|---|---|
| | **0** | **1** | **2** |
| **A**ppearance (color) | blue or pale | blue extremities (pink central) | no cyanosis body/ extremities pink |
| **P**ulse (heart rate) | absent | < 100 /min | > 100 /min |
| **G**rimace (reflex irritability) | no response | grimace | cries or actively withdraws |
| **A**ctivity (muscle tone) | limp | some flexion | active motion |
| **R**espiration (breathing effort) | absent | weak crying, hypoventilation | strong cry |

## Expanded APGAR Scoring*

| Comments: | Administration of: | # Minutes | | | | |
|---|---|---|---|---|---|---|
| | | 1 | 5 | 10 | 15 | 20 |
| | **Oxygen** | | | | | |
| | **PPV/NCPAP** | | | | | |
| | **ET Tube** | | | | | |
| | **Chest Compressions** | | | | | |
| | **Epinephrine** | | | | | |

*Expanded APGAR Scoring is recommended by the American Academy of Pediatrics and the American College of Obstetricians and Gynecologists, 2006

## ▨ **Respiratory Assessment**

Normal Respiratory Rate is 30-60 breaths/min

An irregular breathing pattern does not necessarily indicate a problem

**Periodic Breathing:** common finding with premature babies characterized by intermittent respiratory pauses > 5 seconds

**Apnea** (including Apnea of Prematurity):
abnormal finding in which breathing ceases for > 20 seconds, and may be associated with cyanosis, bradycardia, and hypotonia

## Retractions

| Type | | Location |
|------|------|----------|
| **Upper** | **Suprasternal** | mid-neck, above sternum also called "tracheal tug" |
| | **Supraclavicular** | above clavicles |
| | **Intercostal** | between ribs |
| **Lower** | **Substernal** | just below the sternum |
| | **Subcostal** | just below rib cage also called "belly breathing" |

*General Rule:*
- Upper retractions (suprasternal, supraclavicular) may suggest an upper airway obstructive process
- Lower retractions (substernal, subcostal) usually suggest lower airways obstructive process

## ▓ Neonatal Vitals

| Temperature | 36.5 - 37.0 C |
|---|---|
| HR | 120-160   beats per minute (bpm)<br>100   when asleep<br>180   irregular when crying |
| RR | 30-60   breaths/min |
| BP | $\dfrac{60\text{-}80}{40\text{-}45}$   mm Hg<br>mm Hg (mean = 50) |
| $SpO_2$* | 95% (preterm) - 97% (full term)<br>maintain at roughly 90-95% in<br>preterm infants |

*Transient changes less important than sustained
desaturations, or desaturations with accompanying
bradycardia (HR < 100/min)

Maintain targeted pre-ductal $SpO_2$ after birth per
Neonatal Resuscitation guidelines (see pg 1-4)

## ▓ Auscultation

- Auscultation often occurs at coordinated hands-on time
  with the baby unless clinically indicated by a change in
  status.
- Begin by auscultating the heart.  Murmurs are often easily
  picked up during auscultation.
- Listen for symmetry, comparing the left and right side.
  It may be difficult to differentiate specific lung lobes.
  Sounds transmit from one region to another.

## ▇ Abnormal Pulses and Common Causes

| Type | Possible Cause(s) |
|------|-------------------|
| **Absent (in legs)** | Coarctation of the aorta |
| **Weak** | Dehydration<br>Hypovolemia<br>Shock |
| **Weak**<br>*(with slow upstroke)* | Aortic stenosis<br>Coarctation of the aorta<br>Congestive cardiomyopathy |
| **Bounding pulse**<br>*(rapid and strong)* | ↑ ICP<br>PDA<br>Systemic A-V fistula<br>Anemia<br>Aortic insufficiency<br>Hyperthyroidism (Graves' Disease) |
| **Pulsus alternans**<br>*(regular rhythm, alternating strong and weak beats)* | Myocardial failure |
| **Pulsus paradoxus**<br>*(weak on inspiration, strong on exhalation)*<br><br>***MEDICAL EMERGENCY*** | Cardiac tamponade<br>Constrictive pericarditis<br>Pericardial effusion<br>Severe RDS<br>Severe air trapping |
| **Dicrotic**<br>*(double pulse; strong/weak)* | Fever<br>Preeclampsia |
| **Pulsus bigeminus**<br>*(2 beats close together/coupled)* | PVCs |

## ▨ As, Bs, Ds

While informal, it is common practice to refer to As, Bs and Ds in the NICU. It can be a valuable form of reporting key events during hand-off.

| As | **Apneas** <br> generally cessation of breathing <br> > 20 second/episode |
|----|----|
| Bs | **Bradycardias** <br> HR < 100/min, regardless of time |
| Ds | **Desaturations (SpO$_2$)** <br> Highly variable.  Most clinicians allow for both the severity (i.e. < 70%) and duration (i.e. 20 seconds).  Brief desaturations with spontaneous recovery are seldom reported |

**For example:**

*Baby Jackson had multiple As and Bs today.  He usually responds well to stimulation, but required bagging and chest compressions during one prolonged episode this morning.*

### STUDENT tip

If you are more accustomed to adult critical care, you may feel like you have stepped into a foreign world. Generally speaking, premature babies have lots of variation in their SpO$_2$. Constantly altering the FiO$_2$ can be an endless activity and may increase the risk of oxygen toxicity. So what do we watch for?

Too Low: The length of desaturations and whether bradycardia is present (HR < 100/min) are very important.

Too High: Of equal importance in the NICU (especially with premies) is hyperoxia, or when the SpO$_2$ is sustained above the target range.

## ■ Neonatal Blood Gases

| | Scalp Blood | | | | Cord Blood | | Arterial Blood | | | | |
|---|---|---|---|---|---|---|---|---|---|---|---|
| **Indications** | FHR < 100 or > 160 bpm (Persistent or recurring) Presence of meconium | | | | Ominous FHR Apgar < 7 Wt < 1500 gm Meconium Intrapartum distress Early distress | | Apgar < 7 Post partum distress Early neonatal distress | | | | |
| | Early labor | Mid-labor | Full cerv dil. | Before delivery | Umbilical artery | Umbilical vein | 4 min. | 8 min. | 16 min. | 32 min. | 64 min. |
| **Normal Values** pH | 7.30 | 7.30 | 7.28 | 7.26 | 7.24 | 7.32 | 7.20 | 7.24 | 7.30 | 7.32 | 7.36 |
| $P_{CO_2}$ | 45 | 45 | 49 | 50 | 48 | 38 | 46 | 40 | 35 | 35 | 34 |
| $P_{O_2}$ | 20 | 21 | 19 | 17 | 18 | 28 | 53 | 62 | 68 | 70 | 70 |
| Base def. | 6 | 5 | 6 | 7 | 9 | 7 | 10 | 9 | 8 | 6 | 4 |
| **Clinical Notes** | Taken before birth Capillary puncture is performed on fetal scalp (or presenting part) via endoscope up vaginal canal | | | | Within 15 minutes after birth | | Arterial puncture or arterial line sampling | | | | |

# Systematic Approach to Interpreting a Neo CXR

1. **Confirm patient.**
2. **Confirm date and time.**
3. **Identify type:** AP or PA (special: lateral decubitis)
4. **Check quality:** about 4 vertebrae visible, Inspiratory Film?
   Exp film may show abnorm ↑ heart size, ↓ volume, ↑ interstitium
5. **Check rotation:** clavicles centered around vertebrae
6. **Systematically explore from Outside-to-Inside:**

| | |
|---|---|
| **Soft Tissue** | Amount of tissue<br>Subcutaneous emphysema (crepitus)<br>Gastric Bubble and Liver Size |
| **Bones** | Ribs - splaying (horizontal) = hyperinflation?<br>Obvious spinal deformity (kyphosis, etc.)?<br>Fractures (birth-related injuries - clavicles, etc.) |
| **Heart** | Size: > 60% of thoracic width = abnormal[1]<br>Identify: Major structures (ventricles, etc.) |
| **Lungs** | Expansion (> 6 ribs anterior = hyperinflation)<br>Find trachea, carina (midline?)<br>Find fissures, if visible<br>Find hila (L is above R)<br>Costophrenic and Cardiophrenic Angles<br>   (blunted ~fluid?)<br>Diaphragm: Right is slightly ↑ than Left (liver)<br>             Elevated? Flattened (air trap)?<br>Parenchyma:<br>  Haziness (~atelctasis)<br>  Consolidation (air bronchograms at periphery)<br>  Infiltrates (consolidation, localized or diffuse)<br>  Pneumothorax (lack of vasc. markings)<br>  General abnormalities |
| **Tubes Lines** | ET Tube (~2 cm above carina, often T1-T2)<br>Trach Tube (present or not)<br>NG Tube (projected over stomach)<br>Chest tube(s)<br>EKG leads<br>UAC: dips into pelvis. Tip > T6-T9 or < L2-L5<br>UVC: 0.5 - 1 cm above diaphragm |

# Respiratory Distress

## ■ Silverman Score (Respiratory Distress)

The Silverman/Anderson score is used to assess the degree of respiratory distress in neonates. Scoring ranges from 0 (no distress) to 10 (severe distress).

Used with permission from Silverman, W., and Anderson, D. Pediatrics 17:1, 1956. Copyright American Academy of Pediatrics.

**Interpretations:**

In general:

&lt; 3    Normal, or mild distress

4-6    Moderate respiratory distress

&gt; 6    Impending or established respiratory failure

## Differential Diagnosis of Respiratory Distress (by Acute Sign)

Key
+ Usually Present
++ Nearly Always Present
Arrows indicate decreased or increased

| Sign | Apnea | Asphxia | Bacterial Pneumonia | Choanal Atresia | Congenital Diaphragmatic Hernia | Maternal Drugs | Meconium Aspiration | Pneumothorax | Respiratory Distress Syndrome | Transient Tachypnea of Newborn |
|---|---|---|---|---|---|---|---|---|---|---|
| Breath sounds | → | → | → | | | | → | → | → | |
| Wheezing | | | | | | | | | | |
| RR | | | ← | | ← | → | ← | ← | ← | ← |
| Stridor | | | | + | | | | | | |
| Retractions | | | ++ | ++ | | | ++ | + | ++ | + |
| Nasal Flaring | | | ++ | | | | | + | ++ | |
| Grunting | | | ++ | | | | | + | ++ | |
| ↓ Muscle Tone | | ++ | | | | ++ | + | | | |
| Cyanosis | + | ++ | ++ | ++ | ++ | + | + | ++ | ++ | |
| ↓ HR | ++ | ++ | | | | + | | | | |
| Apnea | ++ | ++ | | + | | + | + | | | |

Neonatal

Assessment

## ◼ Neurological Assessment

Current evidence supports maintaining a minimal stimulation environment (lights, noise, touch) for premature neonates. This includes scheduled times for routine hands-on care whenever possible (called "grouping of care").

There is evidence to suggest that over-stimulation may result in decreased cognitive development. In addition, overexposure to light, noise, or touch may cause physiologic stress (including decompensation in vital signs requiring interventions and possibly increase length of stay).

### The Respiratory Therapist should:

- Minimize routine touch of high-risk neonates, coordinating care with the bedside nurse
- Minimize preventable noise, such as by responding quickly to ventilator alarms, keeping a quite voice volume, etc.
- Help with supportive activities such as ensuring neonate is swaddled when clinically possible

### Altered Neuro Status (in neonates > 28 weeks gestation)

| Term | Description |
|------|-------------|
| **Normal** | Awake<br>Normal arousal/stimulus |
| **Mild Stupor** | Sleepy<br>Slightly diminished arousal/stimulus responses |
| **Moderate Stupor** | Unresponsive<br>Moderate or ↓ arousal/stimulus responses |
| **Deep Stupor** | Unresponsive<br>Absent arousal responses<br>Diminished stimulus response |
| **Coma** | Unresponsive<br>Absent arousal/stimulus response |

Diseases

## CONTENTS

**Other Disease and Disorder with Pulmonary Implications**

# Explanation of Key Used in this Chapter

| NAME - MOST COMMONLY ACCEPTED MEDICAL TERM LISTED IN ALPHABETICAL ORDER (OTHER NAMES OR ABBREVIATIONS) | |
|---|---|
| **Def** | **Definition** of disease/disorder and relevant terminology |
| **Types** | When present, contains information regarding various types of the disease/disorder |
| **Etiology** | **Origin** of disease or disease-causing organisms. |
| **CM** | **Clinical Manifestations** <br> Listings indicate the most commonly found pulmonary [manifestations (not all-inclusive). Manifestations of other body systems are generally not included. |
| **CXR** | **Chest X-Ray** <br> common findings, if relevant. See CXR interpretation in pediatric assessment as well |
| **EBG** | When available, national and international guidelines will be referenced here. |
| **Tx** | **Treatment Overview** <br> including relevant algorithms based on latest evidence-based support |

**Not every category will be presented for every disease - only those that are considered clinically relevant.**

| AIR LEAK SYNDROMES | |
|---|---|
| **Def** | A general term for when air escapes from the lungs and enters any space outside of the alveoli/airways.

This may be in the thoracic space (pneumothorax), around the heart (pneumopericardium), in the interstitial tissues and lymphatic system of the lungs (pulmonary interstitial emphysema), or air in the mediastinal space (pneumomediastinum) |
| **Types** | **See each disorder on following pages for more details:**
• Pneumomediastinum
• Pneumopericardium
• Pneumothorax
• Pulmonary interstitial emphysema (PIE) |
| **Etiology** | **Often secondary to air-trapping, or caused by:**
• Chemical injury
• Trauma
• Surgery
• Iatrogenic (needle puncture, tracheal suction, intubation, mechanical ventilation settings)
• Valsalva maneuvers
• Spontaneous (meconium, transient tachypnea)

**Risk Factors:**
• Underlying lung conditions (RDS, etc.)
• ↓ gestational age = ↑ risk
• Mechanical ventilation (esp ↑ PIP and/or $V_T$) |
| **CM** | Vary depending on severity and location of leak.
See individual disorders (types) on next pages for more details. |
| **Tx** | Vary depending on severity and location of leak.
See individual disorders (types) on next pages for more details. |

Air Leak Disorders (Summary of Manifestations and Treatments)

| Disorder | Clinical Manifestations | Chest X-Ray | Treatment |
|----------|------------------------|-------------|-----------|
| Pneumomediastinum | Asymptomatic-to-severe<br>Distant heart sounds | Air in mediastinum<br>"Spinnaker Sail" sign | None needed most of the time<br>↓ vent volumes/mPaw[1]<br>US-guided percutaneous drainage |
| Pneumopericardium | Asymptomatic-to-severe<br>Distant heart sounds<br>↓ BP<br>↑ HR (initial), then ↓ HR<br>Weak pulses, ↓ Pulse Press<br>Cyanosis<br>↑ RR | Radiolucent area<br>(darker area)<br>encircling heart | **Asymptomatic:**<br>↓ vent volumes/mPaw (if appropriate)[1]<br>Observe closely<br>**Symptomatic:**<br>Immediate needle aspiration<br>Pericardiocentesis (then CXR) if critical<br>Pericardial tube (if it recurs) |
| Pneumothorax | Respiratory distress (sudden)<br>↑ RR<br>↑ HR (initial), then ↓ HR<br>↓ Chest movement<br>Asymmetric chest rise<br>↓ Breath sounds | **Affected Side:**<br>Hyperlucent (no vascular markings)<br>↓ diaphragm<br>Shift of mediastinum away from | Transilluminate (see pg 5-7)<br>**If small/asymptomatic:**<br>Observe closely<br>Supplemental O₂ (for adequate SpO2 only)<br>Needle aspirate (tension, severe)<br>Consider chest tube (tension, severe) |
| Tension (Pneumos - any of above) | Life-threatening symptoms: ↓ HR, ↓ BP, apnea<br>Cardiac Arrest | | TREAT IMMEDIATELY (see txs in red above)<br>Do not wait for CXR confirmation |

| Disorder | Clinical Manifestations | Chest X-Ray | Treatment |
|----------|------------------------|-------------|-----------|
| Pulmonary Interstitial Emphysema (PIE) | Sudden clinical deterioration<br><br>Sudden ABG deterioration<br><br>1st few days of life (usually)<br><br>May be associated with pneumothorax, RDS | Multiple small linear streaks and/or Cysts/Blebs<br><br>Review versus:<br><br>Air bronchograms | **Goal: Supportive, Prevent Damage**<br><br>↓ ventilator volumes (↓ mPaw) if approp.[1]<br><br>Consider HFJV or HFOV<br><br>Minimize ET suction, bagging<br><br>Place involved lung down<br><br>Consider independent lung ventilation<br><br>Consider lobectomy |

[1] Reducing mPAW (mean airway pressure) should be done when clinically appropriate. Options include:

- Decrease set tidal volume (Vt) in volume-targeted modes
- Decrease peak inspiratory pressure (PIP) in pressure-limited modes (including pressure support as needed)
- Decrease positive end expiratory pressure (PEEP) cautiously as it may result in derecruitment of healthy lung units
- Decrease inspiratory time (Ti)
- FiO$_2$ may need to be increased due to the loss of mean airway pressure (mPAW)

**A more complete discussion of ventilator strategies can be found in Chapter 4**

3-6

## AIRWAY ABNORMALITIES
### (UPPER AIRWAY OBSTRUCTIONS)

**Def**

An abnormality or condition in which an obstruction above the small bronchi can result in difficult ventilation.

The normal neonatal airway is smaller, more anterior, and most narrow at around the cricoid. The tongue takes up a larger percentage of the oral cavity as well. Neonates are obligate nose breathers (though they can breathe some through mouth when necessary).

**Types**

| Nose | Trachea/Bronchi | Larynx |
|------|-----------------|--------|
| Choanal atresia | Malacia | Epiglottitis |
| Upper respiratory | Stenosis | floppy |
| infections | Croup | Subglottic stenosis |
| Burns | Lobar emphysema | Laryngospasm |
| Tubes/tape | Tracheal atresia | Laryngeal web |
| | | Cord paralysis |

| Mouth/Pharynx | Extrinsic | Other |
|---------------|-----------|-------|
| Hypoplastic | Goiter | Foreign body |
| mandible | Vascular ring | airway |
| Tongue | Mediastinal mass | obstruction |
| enlargement | T-E fistula | |
| (Down syndrome) | T-I fistula | |
| Pierre-Robin | | |
| Sequence | | |
| Diptheria | | |
| Tonsilitis | | |
| Cysts | | |

TI: Tracheoinnominate  TE: Tracheoesophageal

**Etiology**

Often congenital, though causes vary

**CM**

Variable, but in general range from asymptomatic all the way up through life-threatening (varies based on how much of an obstruction there is). Respiratory distress (tachypnea, retractions, grunting, wheezing, nasal flaring, etc.) is common.

**See next page for specific conditions**

## Selected Airway Abnormalities

| Airway Abnormality | Clinical Manifestations | | Treatments |
|---|---|---|---|
| **Choanal Atresia** *obstruction (bone or membrane) between nose and pharynx* | symptoms are better when crying symptoms are worse when feeding | | **To Diagnose:** pass catheter via nares Infant may appear cyanotic at rest, pink when crying |
| | Unilateral: | asymptomatic-apneic | Usually nothing immediate needed |
| | Bilateral: | gasping, stridor, wheeze, resp distress (retractions, flaring), cyanosis | Emergency oral airway Consider intubation or trach (*secure airway*) Rubber nipple with tip cut off (McGovern Nipple) Surgical intervention (stent, manipulation, septoplasty) |
| **Pierre-Robin Sequence** *micrognathia (small jaw) cleft palate large tongue further back* | Snoring-like/raspy breathing Choke/gag with feeding | | Consider intubation or trach (dep. on severity) Consider placement of nasopharyngeal airway (NPA) Prone (esp. during feeding) Surgical intervention (mandible is fractured) |
| **Subglottic Stenosis** *intrinsic narrowing of airway often due to prolonged intubation but may be congenital* | Respiratory distress Stridor $\downarrow PaO_2$, $\uparrow PaCO_2$ Cyanosis Apnea (possible) | | Consider intubation or tracheostomy (as needed) If post-extubation: cool mist, steroids, heliox therapy, racemic epinephrine If congenital: typically improves with growth, may require surgical intervention (laser, dilation, etc.) |

| | (CONGENITAL) DIAPHRAGMATIC HERNIA (CDH) |
|---|---|
| **Def** | Abdominal contents (viscera) are able to pass into (herniate) the chest. |
| **Etiology** | This is a congenital problem where the diaphragm does not develop properly |
| **CM** | Presents quickly (after crying)—or in days (less severe cases)<br>Left-sided is more common (right-sided or bilateral possible)<br>May become complicated by PPHN<br><br>• Asymptomatic-to-severe distress<br>  (depends on degree and timing of herniation)<br>• Absent breath sounds in affected side (bowel sounds?)<br>• Respiratory distress<br>  if severe distress, may worsen with Bag Mask Ventilation<br>• Scaphoid abdomen (Inward-appearing)<br>• Barrel chest<br><br>CDH Syndrome (associated complications): Pulmonary Hypoplasia, Patent Ductus Arteriosus, Patent Foramen Ovale, Malrotation |
| **CXR** | Diagnosis is often made with CXR (or via US prenatally):<br>Bowel (air- or fluid-filled) in chest cavity<br>Lung on affected side is compressed<br>Displacement of heart, unaffected lung is possible |
| **Tx** | Initiate after delivery:<br>• Intubate immediately, then ventilate<br>  (*Bag-Mask will distend intestine and worsen distress*)<br>• Minimize PIP (goal = < 25 mm Hg— permissive<br>                        hypercapnea 45-55 mm Hg okay)<br>• Minimize FIO₂ (PaO₂ goal = 60-80 mm Hg okay)<br>• Replogle tube to low intermittent suction<br>• Adequate BP support (goal = MAP ≥ 50 mm Hg)<br><br>**Surgical Intervention:** if mild, can repair sooner. If more severe, stabilize before surgical intervention.<br><br>**Consider ECMO** (pre- or post-surgery) especially with PPHN<br>**Consider inhaled Nitric Oxide (iNO)** especially with PPHN |

## MECONIUM ASPIRATION SYNDROME (MAS)

| | |
|---|---|
| **Def** | **Meconium:** First fecal matter of a neonate (sterile, usually dark, black-greenish) composed of bile, mucus, epithelial cells. It is not present until the 3rd trimester<br><br>**Meconium Aspiration Syndrome:** Aspiration of meconium before birth or during the first few breaths of birth |
| **Etiology** | **Predisposing Factors:**<br>    *Postmaturity<br>    Small for Gestational Age (SGA)<br>    Fetal distress/stress or acidosis<br>        (prolapsed cord, prolonged labor, etc.)<br>    Fetal hypoxia (causes gasping)<br>    Maternal drug use (cocaine, tobacco)<br>    Maternal hypotension or hypertension / preeclampsia<br>    Oligohydramnios<br>*Most common predisposing factor |
| **CM** | **Vary from asymptomatic-to-severe distress**<br>*(depends on obstruction severity and location)*<br><br>**Respiratory Distress** *(at birth or shortly after birth)*<br> (tachypnea, retractions, nasal flaring, grunting)<br>Cyanosis<br>Accessory muscle use (retractions)<br>Barrel chest (↑ A-P diameter)<br>Auscultation: coarse crackles (rales, rhonchi)<br>*may lead to air leaks (pneumothorax, etc.)* |
| **Diagnosis** | **Suspected:** amniotic fluid is meconium-stained<br>**Diagnosed:** meconium-stained amniotic fluid, respiratory distress, and CXR (see below) |
| **CXR** | Consolidation (usually patchy) from atelectasis<br>Hyperexpansion (flattened diaphragm, splayed ribs, etc.)<br>Pulmonary air leaks (maybe) |

*Treatment is on page 3-12*

# Meconium Aspiration Effects

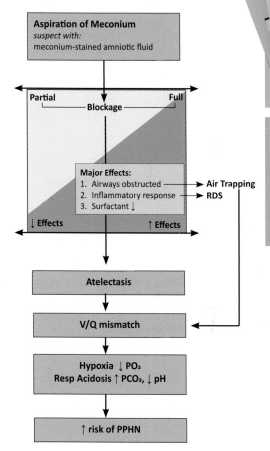

**Aspiration of Meconium**
*suspect with:*
meconium-stained amniotic fluid

Partial ——— **Blockage** ——— Full

**Major Effects:**
1. Airways obstructed → **Air Trapping**
2. Inflammatory response → **RDS**
3. Surfactant ↓

↓ Effects ↑ Effects

Atelectasis

V/Q mismatch

Hypoxia ↓ PO₂
Resp Acidosis ↑ PCO₂, ↓ pH

↑ risk of PPHN

3-11

**Prevent in utero asphyxia**
- Prevent postmaturity

**If evidence of fetal distress (see ch 1)**
- Give oxygen to mother
- Pharmacologic: turn off pitocin, consider tocolytics
- Give volume bolus
- Turn to side
- Immediate delivery?

**Presence of Meconium Pre- and Post-Delivery**

Tx

| | Meconium present at delivery |
|---|---|

*Intrapartum* → **Do NOT Intubate/Suction <u>Trachea</u>[1]**

| Factor | Vigorous | Non-Vigorous |
|---|---|---|
| **Resp. Effort** | Strong | Depressed |
| **Heart Rate** | > 100 bpm | < 100 bpm |
| **Muscle Tone** | Good Tone | Poor Tone |

*Postpartum* → **Do NOT Intubate/Suction <u>Trachea</u>[1]**

Note that suctioning of the mouth/nose is still indicated

**Supportive Care**

The majority of care is now supportive. Note that MAS can lead to Pneumonia, RDS, PPHN (see those sections)

1. Maintain adequate oxygenation
2. Maintain adequate ventilation
   Caution in using N-CPAP in the presence of air-trapping
   Allow adequate exhalation time with air-trapping
   Watch for air leaks (from ball-valve effect)
3. Consider antibiotic administration (prophylactic)
4. Consider surfactant administration
   (meconium deactivates surfactant)

---

[1] Guidelines from American Academy of Pediatrics (AAP), American Heart Association (AHA), and International Liaison Committee on Resuscitation (ILCOR) do NOT recommend <u>tracheal</u> suctioning. Note that mouth/nose should still be suctioned. Rationale is to prevent complications and lack of evidence of better outcomes.

| | PERINATAL B STEPTOCOCCAL (GBS) PNEUMONIA |
|---|---|
| **Def** | A specific infection caused by the bacteria Group B *Streptococcus agalactiae* which may lead to sepsis, pneumonia, or meningitis |
| **Types** | **Early-Onset GBS**: birth-72 hours of life<br>**Late-Onset GBS**: > 72 hours of life |
| **Etiology** | **Early-Onset:** acquired in utero or via passage through vagina<br>**Risk factors include:**<br>• < 37 weeks gestation<br>• Premature rupture of the membranes (PROM)<br>• Maternal fever during labor<br>• Presence of GBS bacteria during pregnancy<br>**Later-Onset acquired:** may be acquired from the mother or other sources |
| **CM** | **Varies in intensity:**<br>• Fever<br>• Difficulty feeding<br>• Irritability/lethargy<br>• Respiratory distress/cyanosis<br>• Hypotension (and other signs of sepsis) |
| **CXR** | Varies, but consistent with pneumonia (consolidation) |
| **EBG** | **CDC: Guidelines for the Prevention of Perinatal Group B Streptococcal (GBS) Disease** |
| **Tx** | **Prevent:**<br>Pregnant women should be screened for GBS and use of intrapartum antibiotics (prophylactic) for high-risk moms<br><br>**Treat:**<br>Antibiotics<br>Support ventilation and oxygenation<br>Identify and treat shock<br>Monitor closely<br>***May develop into pneumonia, sepsis, or meningitis*** |

Neonatal

Diseases

## PERSISTENT PULMONARY HYPERTENSION OF THE NEWBORN (PPHN)

**Def**

Increased pulmonary vascular resistance (PVR) persisting after birth in term or near-term infants, and not caused by congenital heart disease. PPHN can result in severe hypoxemia due to right-to-left shunting through the patent foramen ovale (PFO) and patent ductus arteriosus (PDA).

<u>Fetal circulation</u> through the pulmonary system is high pressure (so it is in a state of relative pulmonary hypertension). <u>At birth</u> pulmonary blood flow ↑ and pulmonary blood pressure ↓ by about 50% (now low pressure). <u>With PPHN</u> this ↓ in vascular tone does not occur.

**Types**

*Due to:*
Lung Disease (Meconium Aspiration, RDS, Pneumonia)
Hypoplastic vasculature (CDH, Pleural Effusion)
Idiopathic (unknown, but possibly due to vascular abnorm.)

**Etiology**

1. **Primary pulmonary vasoconstriction**
   (chronic intrauterine hypoxia or idiopathic)
2. **Secondary to:**
   *Perinatal hypoxia/asphyxia/acidosis*
     Fetal HR abnormalities
     Presence of meconium
     Exposure to SSRI drugs
   *Neonatal* (1st 24-hrs usually)
     Meconium Aspiration Syndrome (MAS)
     Pneumonia and/or Respiratory Distress Syndrome
     Congenital diaphragmatic hernia (CDH)
     Pulmonary hypoplasia

**CM**

**Symptoms usually appear within the first 24-hrs after birth:**
Severe hypoxia/cyanosis may be present
PaO$_2$ may be < 100 mm Hg even on 100% Oxygen
Sudden changes in color (pink ↔ cyanotic)
Mild-Moderate respiratory distress (tachypnea, retractions)
Hypoxia and distress worsens with crying, stress, agitation
Metabolic acidosis
ECHO: ↑ PAP, may be greater than systemic pressures
Cardiovascular: hypotension, Systolic murmur, S2 - loud, ?CHF

| | |
|---|---|
| **Diagnosis** | **Rule out Congenital Heart Disease and Pulmonary Disease** *(severe pulmonary disease can mimic PPHN, or in addition to)*<br><br>**Confirmation usually by echocardiogram (2D):**<br>Confirm R-L Shunting<br>Rule out parenchymal lung disease (RDS, MAS)<br>Rule out Congenital Heart Disease (CHD)<br><br>**Diagnostic Options:**<br>1. Pre- and Post-ductal $SpO_2$ (to show R-L shunt)<br>   Simultaneous measurement at right radial/temporal (pre-ductal) and umbilical or lower extremity (post-ductal).<br>2. Perform echocardiogram<br>3. If echocardiogram is not available, infant should be transferred to a center that can perform this diagnostic evaluation<br><br>**Hyperoxia tests are not currently recommended due to the dangers of hyperoxia in infants. Hyperventilation should not be done due to the danger of cerebral ischemia caused by hypocarbia.** |
| **CXR** | **May be normal** *(still use to rule out other causes)*<br>↓ pulmonary vasculature<br>   (primary pulmonary vasoconstriction)<br>Hyperinflation (possibly)<br>Cardiomegaly<br>Pulmonary parenchymal disease (e.g. RDS, MAS) |
| **Tx** | **Correct or Treat any Secondary Causes (see etiology)**<br>***Promote normal neonatal circulation***<br>*(Goal: ↓ PVR, Reverse R-L Shunt)*<br>• Minimal hands-on (agitation, crying → constriction):<br>   • No heelsticks or punctures (use A-Line, $SpO_2$)<br>   • Delay routine weighing and care<br>   • Minimal auscultation<br>   • CPT and suction only if indicated<br>     (use 2 people to suction)<br>   • Use analgesia/sedation to minimize agitation<br><br>Continued next page |

***Oxygen Therapy*** *(oxygen is a potent pulmonary vasodilator)*
- Monitor pre- and post-ductal $SpO_2$ (see previous page)
- Administer $O_2$ to keep $PaO_2$ consistently > 60 mm Hg
- Wean $FIO_2$ slowly. If $PaO_2$ is labile, keep
  > 100-120 mm Hg. Dramatic changes in $PaO_2$ may occur
  with agitation or rapid weaning
- Consider prone position

***Mechanical Ventilation*** *(supports oxygenation, ventilation)*
Indication: pH < 7.25 with $PaCO_2$ > 55-60 mm Hg
$\qquad\qquad$ $PaO_2$ < 70 mm Hg on $FIO_2$ > 60 mm Hg

*Gentle Ventilation Strategy (normal or mild hypercapnia)*
Goal: pH ≥ 7.25, $PaCO_2$ 40-50 mm Hg, $PaO_2$ > 60 mm Hg
$\quad$ *Avoid dyssynchrony (worsens hypoxemia)*
$\quad$ Mode: volume-targeted ventilation
$\qquad\qquad$ HFOV if on iNO may be preferable
$\quad$ VT: start at 5 cc/kg, avoid VT > 6 cc/kg
$\quad$ Avoid over-expansion (↑ PVR, worsens R-L shunt)

*Weaning*
1. Wean $FIO_2$ slowly to keep $PaO_2$ consistently
   > 60 mm Hg (100-120 mm Hg if baby is labile)
2. Keep VT 4-6 cc/kg, PEEP as needed
3. Wean rate as tolerated

*Weaning too rapidly (allowing $PaCO_2$ > critical level or*
*$PaO_2$ < 100 mm Hg) may result in vasoconstriction and is*
*difficult to reverse.*

### Additional Therapies

If $PaO_2$ remains < 60 mm Hg despite the above therapies, then the following could be considered:

1. Surfactant administration if MAS

2. High Frequency Ventilation if $V_T$ > 6 cc/kg needed, or $PaCO_2$ > 50 on rate of 60/min
   Initial Settings:
   Bias flow: 10-20 L/min (sufficient to deliver mPAW)
   Frequency: 8-10 hz
   Ti: 33%
   Paw: start at 2-3 cmH₂O above current MAP
   ΔP: visible chest wiggle (keep $PaCO_2$ 40-50 mm Hg)
   SEE HFOV (pg 4-67)

3. Inhaled Nitric Oxide *(iNO is a selective pulm. vasodilator)*
   Consider when:
   Oxygen Index > 15 and rising
   Evidence of PPHN on ECHO
   Initial: 20 PPM, then wean to 5-10 PPM when FIO₂ < 60
   SEE iNO (pg 5-18)

   $$OI = \frac{mPAW \times FIO_2}{PaO_2}$$

4. Other Pulmonary Vasodilators:
   Sildenafil and Milrinone are common (see pharmacology)
   Consider also when weaning from iNO

5. ECMO. Consider when infant's condition is worsening despite all other interventions (there is no specific OI value used to determine this any longer)
   SEE ECMO (pg 11-42)

6. Vasopressor Support (keep SVR > PVR to ↓ R-L shunting)
   Dopamine (preferred): 5-10 mcg/kg/min cont. IV; titrate
   Dobutamine: 10 mcg/kg/min cont. IV; titrate
   Nitroprusside: 0.4-5 mcg/kg/min cont IV
   Epinephrine: 0.0.5-0.5 mcg/kg/min cont IV

7. Consider Hgb goal of 15-16 g/dL

| | **RESPIRATORY DISTRESS SYNDROME (RDS)** *INFANT RESPIRATORY DISTRESS SYNDROME (IRDS)* *NEONATAL RESPIRATORY DISTRESS SYNDROME* *OLD: HYALINE MEMBRANE DISEASE (HMD)* |
|---|---|
| **Def** | A syndrome (often of prematurity) which is marked by a <u>**lack of adequate surfactant**</u>, resulting in atelectasis and respiratory distress, often severe. Pulmonary hyaline membranes (a membrane-like layer composed of proteins and dead cells) form in the alveoli, impairing their ability to participate in gas exchange. |
| **Etiology** | **Decreased surfactant (sometimes significantly)** **Predisposing Factors:** <br>• Prematurity (↑ risk with ↓ gestational age) <br>• Perinatal asphyxia <br>• Hypoxia <br>• Acidosis <br>• Hypothermia <br>• Hypovolemia <br>• Hypercapnia <br>• Infants of Diabetic Mothers (IDM) <br>• Birth by Cesarean Section (C-section) <br>• Materal hypotension (preeclampsia) <br>• Rh incompatibility |
| **CM** | **Progressive Respiratory Distress (within 2-3 hours of birth):** <br>• Tachypnea (often first sign) and tachycardia <br>• Cyanosis (may not be present initially) <br>• Expiratory grunting (creates PEEP) <br>• Retractions (sternal, subcostal, intercostal) <br>• Nasal flaring <br>• Paradoxical breathing (seesaw respirations) <br>• Apnea (tiring from ↑ WOB) <br>• ↓ CL (may be noted on ventilator with P-V loop) <br>• ↑ $FIO_2$ needs (↓ $PO_2$) <br>• Auscultation: ↓ breath sounds, crackles <br>• ABG: ↓ pH, ↑ $PaCO_2$, ↓ $HCO_3$, ↓ $O_2$ (anaerobic metabolism) |
| **CXR** | Usually bilateral infiltrates (one lung may be worse) with: <br>• Ground glass (reticulogranular) pattern <br>• Air bronchograms (areas of consolidation) <br>• ↑ pulmonary vasculature |

**Prevent (when possible):**
- Delay premature delivery with tocolytics
- If < 34 weeks, promote surfactant production:
  - Administer corticosteroids to mother for 24-48 hours before expected delivery
  - Other treatments have been evaluated, but are not consistent (prolactin, ambroxol, aminophylline, etc.)

**Delivery Room Stabilization**
*Note: distress is not always noted at birth, but may be delayed several hours*
- Initiate N-CPAP in all preterm infants with RDS
- Oxygen: Use targeted pre-ductal $SpO_2$ (see pg 1-4)
- Surfactant: Give within 2 hrs to premature infants if not responding to N-CPAP

**General Management Strategies**
- Administer surfactant (see pg 5-22) as soon as possible if infant is not responding to N-CPAP
- Maintain temperature at 36.5° - 37.5° C (avoid ↑ and ↓)
- Maintain glucose, fluid, electrolytes (avoid fluid overload)
- Maintain BP and Hematocrit (40-45%)
- Minimize handling / stimulation (including suctioning)
- Administer caffeine citrate (↓ apneas and bronchopulmonary dysplasia) to preterm infants

**Ventilation/Oxygen Support Strategies**
- Evidence supports early use of N-CPAP (establishes FRC; N-CPAP alone requires good respiratory effort)
- If infant fails N-CPAP ($FIO_2$ > 0.4 and/or pH < 7.25) then consider noninvasive or invasive ventilation (and surfactant if not administered or if additional dose is appropriate)
- Goal of ventilation is to provide adequate oxygenation and ventilation while protecting the lungs from barotrauma, volutrauma, oxygen toxicity
- Consideration of HFJV or HFOV with same goal as above. Some clinicians use prophylactically (before injury), and others use as a rescue (status is declining) option
- Avoid sustained <u>hypoxemia</u> or <u>hyperoxemia</u>
- Consider sedation if dyssynchrony noted (but may ↓ respiratory drive)

Tx

| | | **TRANSIENT TACHYPNEA OF THE NEWBORN (TTN)** |
|---|---|---|
| | **Def** | Respiratory distress at birth due to 2 major factors:<br>1. Fetal lung fluid is not resorbed<br>2. Pulmonary vascular system fails to immediately transition to low pressure (so a relatively increased PVR) |
| | **Etiology** | • Prematurity<br>• Delayed absorption of fetal lung fluid<br>• Myocardial failure (less common)<br>**Predisposing Factors:**<br>• C-section birth<br>• Over-sedated mothers<br>• Infant of a diabetic mother (IDM)<br>• Maternal asthma<br>• Polycythemia<br>• Asphyxia<br>• Near-term hypotension<br>• Epidural administration |
| | **CM** | **Presents within first day of life (usually within 2-hours)**<br>• Tachypnea (> 60/min)—may be only real sign<br>• ↑ Work of Breathing (tends to be mild)<br>  (nasal flaring, retractions, grunting)<br>• Mild cyanosis<br>• Mild respiratory acidosis with hypoxemia<br>**\*usually self-limiting (resolves in 12-24 hrs, max ~72 hrs)\***<br>**some progress to severe PPHN** |
| | **CXR** | Flattened diaphragms<br>Fluid in fissures<br>Perihilar streaking (prominent vascular markings) |
| | **Tx** | **Supportive:**<br>• Oxygen for hypoxemia (usually < 40%)<br>• N-CPAP for respiratory distress<br>• Consider delay of feeding (to prevent aspiration)<br><br>If extensive support is needed (mechanical ventilation, $FIO_2$ > 60%), consider other possibilities: Group B Strep, RDS, PPHN, Sepsis, Pneumonia |

| CONGENITAL HEART DEFECTS | |
|---|---|

**Def**

An abnormality in the heart that is present at birth

**Types**

**Two Main Types of Defects:**

| Right-to-Left Shunt Cyanotic | Left-to-Right Shunt Acyanotic |
|---|---|
| Low SpO₂/SaO₂ | Normal SpO₂/SaO₂ |
| Blood from right side of heart (not oxygenated) | Blood from left side of heart (oxygenated) |
| Bypasses the lungs (where it is usually oxygenated) | Transfers back to the right side of the heart (increases volume of blood to the lungs and may increase pulmonary pressures, which are supposed to be lower than systemic pressures) |
| And then enters the left side of the heart (still not oxygenated) | |

*Shunts are usually not absolute: some blood may still pass through its normal pathway.*

**Etiology**

Unknown, or may be associated with:
- Chromosomal anomalies
- Congenital syndromes
- Congenital infection
- Infant of a diabetic mother (IDM)
- Maternal drug infection

**CM**

**General:**
- Heart murmur
- Poor feeding/weight gain
- Hypoxemia
- Signs/symptoms of congestive heart failure (CHF)

**Signs and Symptoms of Cardiac Disease in Infants**
- Cry: weak and muffled, loud and breathless
- Cyanotic: usually generalized; ↑ in supine position; often unrelieved by oxygen administration; may worsen with crying; gray; dusky
- Acyanotic: pale, with or without mottling on exertion
- Activity level varies from restless to lethargic
- Posturing (hypotonic, neck hyperextended, knee-chest)

3-21

| | |
|---|---|
| | • Persistent bradycardia (< 120 bpm) or persistent tachycardia ( > 160 bpm)<br>• Respirations: counted when neonate is sleeping to identify the problem early<br>• Tachypnea (> 60 breaths/min)<br>• Retractions with nasal flaring<br>• Dyspnea with diaphoresis or grunting<br>• Gasping followed in 2-3 minutes by respiratory distress (treat promptly)<br>• Chronic cough (not often seen)<br>• Grunting with exertion such as crying or feeding by nipple |
| **CXR** | ↑ or ↓ pulmonary vasculature |
| **Tx** | **Pulse oximetry newborn screening** (mandatory in some states):<br>• Perform after 24 hours of life or as late as possible if early discharge is planned<br>• Recommended in the right hand and either foot.<br>• Positive screening includes one of the following:<br>  • SpO₂ (SaO₂) < 90%<br>  • SpO₂ (SaO₂) < 95% in both upper and lower extremities on 3 measurements, each separated by an hour<br>  • SpO₂ (SaO₂) difference > 3% between upper and lower extremities<br>• Note that a positive test will not necessarily indicate cyanotic CHD, nor will a negative test definitively exclude it<br><br>**Overview** (see following table for specific defects)<br>• Consider oxygen administration<br>• Consider prostaglandins<br>• Consider digitalis/diuretics<br>• Consider corrective surgery<br>• Consider palliative measures |

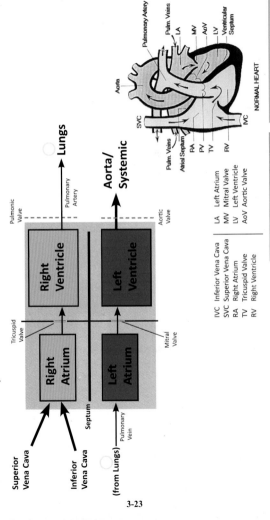

# Congenital Heart Defects

## Acyanotic (Left-to-Right Shunt)

| Defect | Description | Clinical Manifestations | Management |
|---|---|---|---|
| **Aortic Stenosis (AS)** | Obstruction of blood flow from left ventricle to aorta (often due to narrowing of the aortic valve) | Classic triad:<br>• Angina pectoris<br>• Heart failure (paroxysmal nocturnal dyspnea, orthopnea, dyspnea on exertion, SOB)<br>• Syncope (upon exertion) | • Balloon dilation of valve<br>• Aortic valve replacement (severe stenosis) |
| **Atrial Septal Defect (ASD)** | Hole in atrial septum which results in blood flowing between the right and left atrium (right-to-left or left-to-right blood flow can result) | • May be asymptomatic<br>• Right heart failure<br>• Shunt manifestations | May spontaneously close<br>Surgical closure (patch)<br>Catheter |
| **Atrioventricular Septal Defect (AVSD)** | Holes between the right- and left-side chambers of the heart. Valves may not form correctly. Results in excessive blood flow to lungs (leading to congestion). | • Mild cyanosis<br>• ↓ SpO₂<br>• Congestive heart failure<br>• CXR: cardiomegaly with atrial dilation, dilated PA | Diuretics<br>Digoxin (for CHF)<br>Surgical closure (patch) |

| Defect | Description | Clinical Manifestations | Management |
|--------|-------------|-------------------------|------------|
| **Coarctation of the Aorta** | Narrowing of aorta near ductus arteriosus (at the aortic isthmus). It results in the left ventricle having to work harder to push blood through (or, if severe, the left ventricle fails). | • Degree of shunt determines severity<br>• Congestive heart failure<br>• Left ventricle hypertrophy<br>• Lack of palpable pulses in legs, groin<br>• CXR: cardiomegaly | • IV prostaglandin<br>• Mechanical ventilation<br>• Urgent surgical repair |
| **Patent Ductus Arteriosus (PDA)** | Failure of the ductus arteriosus (connects aorta and pulmonary artery) to close. This results in blood flowing from the aorta to the pulmonary artery. | • Systolic murmur<br>• Pulmonary edema<br>• Bounding peripheral pulses<br>• Hypotension<br>• Tachypnea, ↑ WOB | • Small PDA may not require intervention<br>• Indomethacin (premie)<br>• Ibuprofen (caution with premies)<br>• Catheterization closure<br>• Surgical ligation (severe)<br><br>No longer treated with Oxygen |
| **Pulmonary Stenosis (PS)** | Obstruction of blood flow from right ventricle to pulmonary artery. It is caused by a narrowing at one or more points (of pulmon. artery). | • Murmur<br>• Cyanosis (severe stenosis)<br>• Right ventricular failure<br>• Shortness of breath | • Balloon dilation of valve<br>• Surgical correction |

| Defect | Description | Clinical Manifestations | Management |
|---|---|---|---|
| **Ventricular Septal Defect (VSD)** | Holes in ventricular septum which results in blood flowing between the right and left ventricles (left-to-right blood flow results) | • May be asymptomatic<br>• Poor eating<br>• Failure to thrive<br>• Tachypnea, Dyspnea<br>• Congestive Heart Failure (severe)<br>• Easy tiring | May spontaneously close (~50%)<br>Surgical closure if symptomatic—usually first year |
| **Cyanotic (Right-to-Left Shunt)** | | | |
| **Hypoplastic Left Heart Syndrome (HLHS)** | All of the structures on the left side of the heart are severely underdeveloped—making it nonfunctional. The aorta is also very small.<br><br>This results in the right ventricle having to handle the load of both sides (PDA is used for systemic circulation). **If the PDA closes, shock follows.** | • Life-threatening shock<br>• Cyanosis<br>• Poor Perfusion<br>• Respiratory distress which worsens as PDA closes<br>• Weak pulses | **Stabilization:**<br>IV prostaglandin (to stop PDA from closing)<br>Avoid O₂ (promotes ↑ blood flow to lungs)<br>Mechanical ventilation?<br>Treat CHF<br><br>**Treatment:**<br>Cardiac transplantation<br>Staged reconstruction |

| Defect | Description | Clinical Manifestations | Management |
|---|---|---|---|
| **Tetralogy of Fallot (TOF)** | 4 Anomalies: pulmonary stenosis, ventricular septal defect, overriding aorta, right ventricular hypertrophy | • SpO₂ usually normal initially<br>• Cyanosis<br>• Systolic ejection murmur<br>• Boot-shaped heart on CXR | • IV prostaglandins<br>• Surgery (patch VSD, resection, enlarge RV outlet path patch) |
| **Total Anomalous Pulmonary Venous Return (TAPVR)** | All 4 pulmonary veins drain to right atrium through abnormal connections; An atrial septal defect is necessary for survival | • May be asymptomatic<br>• Severe cyanosis<br>• Hypotension<br>• Pulmonary edema<br>• PPHN<br>• Respiratory distress | • Surgery<br>• ASD patch<br>• Tie off pulmonary drainage units |
| **Transposition of the Great Arteries (TGA)** | Major vessels switched:<br>• Aorta comes from right ventricle (instead of left ventricle)<br>• Pulmonary artery comes from left ventricle (instead of right ventricle)<br><br>Ventricular septal defect is necessary for survival | • Large, vigorous infant with cyanosis without respiratory distress<br>• Murmur possible<br>• "Egg on a stick" on CXR | • Creation of VSD via emergent balloon septostomy<br>• Surgery (repair ASD/VSD, cut off great vessels and switch/move coronary arteries) |

| Defect | Description | Clinical Manifestations | Management |
|--------|-------------|------------------------|------------|
| **Tricuspid Atresia** | Tricuspid valve (between right atrium and right ventricle) isn't formed. Results in under-developed right ventricle | • Progressive cyanosis<br>• Tachypnea<br>• Poor feeding | Surgery<br>Fontan procedure |
| **Truncus Arteriosus** | A single blood vessel comes off both right and left ventricles (instead of the normal pulmonary artery + aorta)—usually a result of a ventricular septal defect, resulting in mixing of blood | • Cyanosis<br>• Congestive heart failure<br>• Fatigue/lethargy<br>• Poor feeding<br>• Tachypnea<br>• Digital clubbing | Surgery (Separate PA from truncus, close VSD, create connection for RV and PA via valved conduit) |

| | GASTROSCHISIS/OMPHALOCELE |
|---|---|
| | **A birth defect in which the intestines are outside the body** |
| **Def** | **Gastroschisis:** due to a weakness in the body wall, usually on the right side, intestines are extruded outside the body with no membrane covering |
| | **Omphalocele:** intestines fail to return to the abdomen during development, resulting in their remaining in the umbilical ring (there is a presence of membrane covering, may rupture) |
| **Etiology** | **The cause can be largely unknown, but:** ↓ Maternal Age = ↑ risk of omphalocele/gastroschisis |
| **CM** | Respiratory symptoms vary by size/complexity: • Decreased chest excursion • Respiratory distress |
| **CXR** | Bowel loops on exterior of the body Diaphragm may be ↑ |
| **Tx** | **Prenatal diagnosis can be made using ultrasound** **Delivery Room:** • The bowel should be wrapped with sterile saline dressings and covered with plastic wrap • OG (Replogle tube) should be placed and low intermittent suction used in order to decompress stomach • Ensure a patent airway **Post-Delivery:** Supportive care of respiratory/cardiac status (the need for intervention varies) **Surgical:** • In most cases intestines are placed back in abdominal cavity and cavity is closed • NOTE: A decrease in diaphragmatic excursion and lung compliance will occur upon closure. Too tight of a closure can result in ↑ PIP, ↓ venous return to heart (↓ CO), ↓ GFR • More complex cases may require a staged silo |

## INTRAVENTRICULAR HEMORRHAGE (IVH)

| | | | |
|---|---|---|---|
| **Def** | Bleeding into the fluid-filled areas (ventricles) of the brain, often due to prematurity. | | |

**IVH Grading** (Increased severity = ↑ morbidity/mortality)

| | | |
|---|---|---|
| **Mild** | **Grade I** | Germinal matrix or Germinal matrix + IVH < 10% |
| **Moderate** | **Grade II** | Occupies ≤ 50% of lateral ventricle volume |
| **Severe** | **Grade III** | Occupies > 50% of lateral ventricle volume |
| | **Grade IV** | Parenchymal bleed (any location / amount) |

*(Types)*

**Etiology**

**Most frequently in premature infants (< 1500 g birth wgt)**
- Genetic issues
- Prenatal factors (lack of steroids, etc.)
- Labor and delivery (mode, breech, delayed cord clamping)
- Respiratory distress
- Neonatal resuscitation

**CM**

**Silent:** noted on Ultrasound, but asymptomatic
**Common:** Δ level of consciousness, hypotonia, respiratory function
**Serious:** Stupor/coma, irregular respirations, hypoventilation, apnea, posturing, seizures, fixed pupils

**Tx**

**Prevention:**
- Delay birth when possible
- Administer antenatal corticosteroids
- Delay cord clamping by 30-60 seconds
- Avoid hypo- and hypertension
- Avoid large infusions of fluid
- Manage coagulation abnormalities

**Management:**
↓ further brain injury (cerebral perfusion, oxygenation)
- Maintain adequate perfusion (avoid hypo/hyper tension)
- Provide adequate oxygenation and ventilation
  - Avoid ↓ or ↑ $PCO_2$, ↓ pH

| | **NECROTIZING ENTEROCOLITIS (NEC)** |
|---|---|
| **Def** | Variable damage to the intestinal tract of premature infants (usually weighing < 1500 g). This may be a GI emergency. |
| **Types** | NEC is usually staged as Bell Stages IA, IB, IIA, IIB, IIIA, IIIB. Actual staging is beyond the scope of this text |
| **Etiology** | **Mortality rates are high - 50% or more (premature infants)** <br><br>• Etiology is largely unknown<br>• Lack of oxygen/blood flow to intestines causes weakening<br>• Bacteria enters the intestines, causing damage or death to tissue, with ↑ risk of infection<br>• Poor immune response<br>• Formula feeds |
| **CM** | **Appears 1-3 days after birth, up to several weeks after birth:**<br>• Vomiting<br>• Diarrhea<br>• Abdominal distention / delayed gastric emptying<br><br>**Systemic Signs:**<br>• Apnea<br>• Bloody stools<br>• Lethargy<br>• ↓ peripheral perfusion<br>• Shock (advanced sign)<br>• Cardiovascular collapse<br>• Respiratory failure<br>• Lactic acidosis (↓ CO) |
| **CXR** | Abdominal x-rays are best, but abdominal free air may be noted on CXR (ominous sign) |
| **Tx** | **Treatment is based upon staging:**<br>• Bell Stages IA and IB: NPO x 3 days, TPN, antibiotics<br>• Bell Stages IIA and IIB: Respiratory/Cardiac support, fluid resuscitation, NPO, antibiotics, surgical consult, TPN after stabilized<br>• Bell Stage IIIA: NPO x 14 days, fluid resuscitation, inotropics, ventilator support, surgical consult, TPN after stabilized<br>• Bell Stage IIIB: Surgical intervention |

## NEONATAL ABSTINENCE SYNDROME (NAS)

**Def**

Group of symptoms/problems caused by withdrawal to addictive drugs, either due to maternal use of drugs or discontinuation of drugs (e.g. fentanyl, morphine)

Note that some drugs may not cause withdrawal (e.g. cocaine), but may remain in the infant's system for several days.

**General Withdrawal Symptoms**
- High-pitched cry
- Restlessness (dys-synchrony on ventilator)
- Tremors/seizures
- Fever
- Vomiting/diarrhea
- Other: Tolerance to some drugs may develop (opioids), diminishing response to administered drugs in NICU

**Selected Drugs consistent with withdrawal symptoms[1]**

**CM**

| Drug | Significant Signs | Onset | Duration |
|------|-------------------|-------|----------|
| Alcohol | Seizures | 3-12 hr | 18 mos |
| Barbiturates | Severe tremors Vasomotor instability | 1-14 d | 4-6 mos |
| Caffeine | Bradycardia Tachypnea | birth | 1-7 days |
| Diazepam | Hypothermia Apnea Hypertonia Tachypnea | hours-wks | 8 mos |
| Opioids Benzo-diazepines | Tolerance Wakefulness Seizures | < 1 d (or delayed) | 1 wk |
| SSRIs | Tachypnea Hypoglycemia Seizures | hours-days | 1-4 wk |

**Delivery Room**
- Do not use naloxone if known opioid dependency (abrupt withdrawal may cause seizures)

**Management**
- Treatment is largely supportive
- Minimize environmental stimuli
- Careful swaddling (avoids autostimulation)
- Promote adequate rest and sleep
- Provide sufficient caloric intake for weight gain
- Effects on mechanical ventilation vary depending on a number of factors (type of drug, amount of drug, frequency of drug, and metabolic/distribution issues).
  - Dyssynchrony is likely with tachypnea, restlessness, seizures
  - Spontaneous modes may be challenging with apneas, lethargy
  - Sedation needs to be viewed in the context of tolerance

Consider use of pharmacology in more complex cases (seizures present, dehydration by vomiting or diarrhea, poor weight gain)

Tx

[1] Adapted from the American Academy of Pediatrics. Hudak ML, Tan RC. Neonatal Drug Withdrawal. Pediatrics 2012.

| NEONATAL APNEA |
| :---: |
| (APNEA OF PREMATURITY / PERIODIC BREATHING) |

**Def** Cessation of breathing due to immaturity of respiratory control. May be central (neuro), obstructive (anatomical), or mixed.

**Types**

Apnea of Prematurity versus Periodic Breathing

| | Apnea of Prematurity[1] | Periodic Breathing |
| :--- | :--- | :--- |
| Normal in Prematurity? | No | Yes |
| Age | < 37 weeks gestation | Up to 6 mos age |
| Cycles | No | Alternating breaths and brief respiratory pauses |
| Apnea period | > 20 seconds < 20 seconds if desaturation or bradycardia | 5-10 seconds |
| Interventions | Often requires interventions (see Tx) | Rarely required |

[1] a separate disorder exists for those > 37 weeks (Apnea of Infancy)

**Etiology**

APNEA OF PREMATURITY
**Prematurity:** incomplete development of neurological drive to breathe
**Sepsis:** serious cause, rule out first
There are many other causes of apneas in neonates/infants besides prematurity, including hypoxia, RDS, airway obstructions, vagal stimulation, drugs (maternal or neonatal), and CNS dysfunction.

**Tx**

Apnea of Prematurity:
**Pharmacologic Management:** The use of a methylxanthine is strongly recommended (caffeine citrate is common) which acts as a neurologic stimulant for breathing. See Pharmacology chapter for details.

## Neonatal Apnea Intervention Algorithm

Apnea[1]

← Observe

← Stimulate[2]

Positive Pressure Ventilation[3]

← Chest Compressions/ Neonatal Resusc.

Stop Intervention and Wean F$_I$O$_2$ Rapidly when Stable (HR and SpO$_2$)

SpO$_2$

HR

60

[1] Generally, interventions are not employed until symptomatic (SpO$_2$ drops severely and/or sustained, then cardiac involvement). Consider reversible causes of apnea, including vagal stimulation, respiratory arrest (secretions, etc.), airway obstruction, drugs, or CNS dysfunction.

[2] Provide gentle but firm tactile stimulation: flick sole of foot, rub legs, chest or back. Do not inflict pain.

[3] Use same FIO$_2$ as infant was on before event, or ↑ at small intervals (no more than 3-4% at a time)

## NEONATAL ENCEPHALOPATHY[1]

**Def**

Altered neurological function in an infant ≥ 35 weeks gestation which results in an altered LOC, seizures, respiratory compromise, and depression of tone/reflexes

**Types**

**Hypoxic-Ischemic Encephalopathy (HIE)**
a type of neonatal encephalopathy marked by contributing events near the time of labor and delivery. Look for the following:

- APGAR < 5 at 5 min and 10 min
- Umbilical Artery pH < 7.0 (acidemia)
- Neuroimaging evidence of Acute Brain Injury
- Presence of Multi-System Organ Failure (renal, hepatic, hematologic, cardiac, metabolic, gastrointestinal)
- Major Hypoxic or Ischemic event
- Abnormal FHR

**CM**

**Categories of Neonatal Encephalopathy**

|  | Mild | Moderate | Severe |
|---|---|---|---|
| **LOC** | Hyperalert | Lethargic | Stuporous |
| **Tone** | Normal | Hypotonia | Flaccid |
| **Reflexes** | Normal | Decreased | Absent |
| **Seizures** | None | Possible | Likely |
| **Morbidity** | None | Long-term neurological disabilties | |

Adapted from *Pediatric Annals* 17:8, 1998

**Tx**

- Therapeutic hypothermia x 72 hours (33-35° C) for term or later preterm
- Maintain adequate ventilation and oxygenation
  If PPHN also, treat aggressively to maintain adequate oxygenation
- Maintain adequate hemodynamics (avoid hypo/hyper)
- Maintain fluid balance (no fluid overload)
- Treat underlying causes and complications

[1]Adapted and summarized from: Report of the American College of Obstetricians and Gynecologists' Task Force on Neonatal Encephalopathy. Pediatrics 2014.

| TRACHEOESOPHAGEAL FISTULA (TEF) | |
|---|---|
| **Def** | Abnormal passage between the trachea and esophagus |
| **Types** | **Presence of Esophageal Atresia[1] (EA)**<br>95% of the time<br>Immediately symptomatic (see CM below)<br><br>**Absence of Esophageal Atresia[1]:**<br>Large fistula: symptomatic (see CM below)<br>Small fistula (H-Type): minimally symptomatic, or undetected<br>　may display mild respiratory distress with feeding<br>　may have recurrent pneumonia |
| **Etiology** | Usually congenital, though may be caused if using a cuffed ET Tube (unusual with neonates, but possible) |
| **CM** | **THREE C's: Choking, Coughing, Cyanosis**<br>• Excess salivation<br>• Aspiration<br>• Gastric distention<br>• Tracheal compression/deviation |
| **Tx** | **Diagnosis of EA**: Attempt to pass a catheter into stomach. If catheter doesn't go beyond 10-15 cm, TEF should be suspected. Confirm with CXR which will show curling of catheter.<br><br>• Place nasogastric tube as soon as fistula is identified<br>• Nothing by mouth: provide parenteral nutrition<br>• Position for optimal airway patency and ventilation<br>• Aspirate secretions from oropharynx and pouch<br>• Prevent aspiration<br>• Surgical correction (ligation)<br><br><u>Note</u>: CPAP is relatively contraindicated as it may cause gastric distension |

[1]**Esophageal Atresia (EA):** congenital disorder where the esophagus fails to develop fully as a continuous passage

Neonatal

Ventilation

CONTENTS

## Some Notes About This Chapter

### Terms/Abbreviations Used

| mPAW | **Mean Airway Pressure** |
|------|--------------------------|
|      | We have decided on this abbreviation as it is easy to differentiate from any other abbreviation. Other acceptable abbreviations include MAP (also Mean Arterial Pressure), $\overline{Paw}$, $\overline{Paw}$. |
| FIO₂ | **Oxygen Percentage** |
|      | $FIO_2$ by definition is a decimal equivalent of the fractional inspired oxygen. It is more clinically relevant to set $O_2$ by %, so you will see $FIO_2$ used as a % in this chapter. |

**Special Note:**
This chapter was created based upon hundreds of hours of research and collaboration. It is important to note that clinical practice should be evidence-based. Where evidence may be lacking or unavailable, best and current clinical practice should be referenced.

As with all resources, there is no subsitution for systematic assessment skills and solid critical thinking.

**Modes/Therapeutic Modalities are presented throughout the chapter with a letter beside the title. These coordinate with the lists of modes at the beginning of each section.**

## ■ General Considerations

### Neonatal Physiology Affecting Ventilation

- Higher-than-normal chest wall compliance
  *Excessive inspiratory efforts will collapse the upper airway, lungs*
- Horizontal ribs and flatness of diaphragm
  *Reduces potential lung expansion and resulting tidal volumes*
- Possible right-to-left shunting
  *Patent Ductus Arteriosus (PDA) and/or*
  *Patent Foramen Ovale (PFO)*
- Possible left-to-right shunting
  *Increases risk of pulmonary edema, usually via PDA*
- Insufficient collateral ventilation between alveoli
  *Increased risk of atelectasis and airway closure*
- Surfactant deficiency
  *Results in ↓ Compliance, ↓ FRC, baby may grunt/shorten expira-*
  *tory time to maintain FRC*
- Postnatal clearance of lung liquid
  *Increased amounts of interstitial fluid*
- High metabolic rate
- Less muscle mass, muscle fibers, and ↓ oxidative capacity

### Other Neonatal Considerations

- There are no well-defined absolute criteria for whether to initiate noninvasive or invasive mechanical ventilation for neonates/infants
- Consider everything in context of physiology and pathophysiology
- Consider early intubation/mechanical ventilation when:
  - Congenital anomalies affect ventilatory function
    (congenital diaphragmatic hernia should always be intubated)
  - Infant has low APGAR scores and responds poorly to resuscitation efforts
  - Infant has severe sepsis or compromised pulmonary blood flow (PPHN)
  - Progressive atelectatic disease is evident
  - Breathing is labored and/or blood gases show progressive hypoxemia or hypercarbia

# Ventilation Overview

*Due to recent evidence supporting improved outcomes (inlcuding de-creased rates of BPD), many clinicians show restraint in utilizing invasive mechanical ventilation strategies, resulting in more use of noninvasive strategies. When invasive strategies are employed, neonates are often weaned quickly, often transitioning to noninvasive support.*

## ◼ Mechanical Ventilation

### Indications for Mechanical Ventilation

- <u>Apnea</u>: prolonged or repetitive, unresponsive apnea associated with bradycardia and/or cyanosis
- <u>Respiratory failure in newborns</u>:
  - $PaO_2 < 50$ mm Hg (or persistent $SpO_2 < 85\%$ on $FiO_2 \geq 60\%$
  - $PaCO_2$ persistently > 60-65 mm Hg
    ( > 55 mm Hg in infants < 1500 g or < 2 wks of age)
  - pH < 7.20
- <u>Impending respiratory failure</u>. While somewhat subjective, the following should be considered:
  - Worsening oxygenation
  - Respiratory distress ($\uparrow$ RR > 60 breaths/min with retractions, grunting, nasal flaring)
  - ABG values may or may not be within acceptable ranges

### Contraindications for Mechanical Ventilation

- < 22 weeks gestation or birth weight < 400 g
- Congenital anomalies incompatible with survival (anacephaly, lethal genetic disorders)
- Severe prolonged Hypoxic-Ischemic Encephalopathy with very poor prognosis

## Noninvasive versus Invasive Strategies

### Five Major Classifications of Neonatal Support
*(Presented in order of support - least to most)*

| | |
|---|---|
| **Low-Flow** | Flows produced as low as ¼ L/min, usually with a blender and flowmeter. Interfaces include Nasal Cannula, Oxygen Tent, etc. See Procedures Chapter. |
| **Nasal CPAP (and CPAP-like effect)** | Short prongs are placed in each nare to create a loose seal, and a pressure is provided from a simple flowmeter or equipment designed to provide CPAP. |
| **Noninvasive Ventilation** | Short prongs are placed in each nare, or a slightly longer catheter is placed 2-3 cm into a single nare where support (at least some of which consists of mandatory breaths) is provided by a number of modes. |
| **Conventional Invasive Ventilation** | Requires invasive endotracheal intubation (or tracheostomy). Varying levels of support (modes) are provided via the ET Tube. |
| **High Frequency Ventilation** | This specialized form of ventilation uses very high rates and low tidal volumes in a lung-protective strategy. |

### STUDENT tip

CPAP applications for infants are applied nasally, which is unlike some adult applications where masks cover the nares and mouth. Why would that be? 1) Neonates are obligate nose-breathers, so there is usually no need to provide CPAP at the mouth; 2) Nasal interfaces decrease the risk of aspiration due to vomiting, and for the risk of abdominal distension.

# ▧ Monitoring

*Careful and consistent bedside monitoring is important, but systematic evaluation and analysis is critical.*

**Continuous Monitoring:**
- Cardiac activity (monitor)
- Carbon dioxide (TcCO$_2$, ETCO$_2$, CBG/VBG/ABG)
- Oxygen delivery (SpO$_2$)
- Proximal airway pressures (PIP, PEEP, mPAW)
- Respiratory Rate
- Tidal Volume (VT) delivery
- I:E ratio (*f*, TI, etc.)

**Periodic Monitoring:**
- Acid-Base (CBG, VBG, ABG)
- Blood Pressure (invasive or noninvasive)
- Chest X-Ray
- Physical asssessment (auscultation, WOB, etc.)

**Conventional Ventilator Parameters Overview**
*Details on the following pages:*

| Parameter | Potential Ranges | |
|---|---|---|
| Tidal Volume (VT) | 4-6 mL/kg | |
| Peak Inspiratory Pressure (PIP) | 15-25 cm $H_2O$ | |
| Mean Airway Pressure (mPAW or $\overline{P}aw$) | 5-15 cm $H_2O$ | |
| Positive End Expiratory Pressure (PEEP) | 4-7 cm $H_2O$ | |
| Frequency (*f*) or Rate | 20-60 breaths/min | |
| I:E Ratio *(dependent on $T_i$)* | 1:1 to 1:3 | |
| | **Premature** | **Term** |
| Inspiratory Time (TI) | 0.25-0.35 sec | 0.3-0.4 sec |
| Inspiratory Flow ($\dot{V}I$) | 5-8 L/min | 6-10 L/min |
| Flow Waveform | Decelerating  Square  Sinusoidal | |
| FIO₂ (O₂%) | **21%** - 100% (lower is better) | |
| Leak Compensation | uses algorithm | |

On the following pages parameters with a blue heading are generally set directly on the equipment (dependent on mode). Parameters with a red heading are important to be aware of, but generally are not set directly.

Neonatal

Ventilation

| Tidal Volume (VT) | |
|---|---|
| **Normal Range** | Low Birthweight: 4-6 mL/kg<br>Term: 5-6 mL/kg |
| **Clinical Notes** | *In the absence of VT measurement, aim for a gentle rise and fall of the chest.*<br><br>*VT is most often measured by:*<br>Delivered tidal volume (VTI)<br>Exhaled tidal volume (VTE) - most common<br>(VT should be measured at ET tube)<br><br>*Note:* VT monitor can measure % leak<br><br>**% leak** = $\dfrac{\text{VT delivered} - \text{VT expired} \times 100}{\text{VT delivered}}$<br><br>A small leak is acceptable and desirable around cuffless ET tubes used in neonates. The presence of a leak suggests tracheal inflammation is minimal. |
| **Cautions** | Use of lower tidal volume to prevent lung over-expansion (volutrauma) must be balanced with overcoming sensor deadspace (~1 cc). |

| Peak Inspiratory Pressure (PIP) | |
|---|---|
| **Average Range** | 15-25 cm $H_2O$ |
| **Clinical Notes** | The lowest PIP that adequately ventilates the patient is usually appropriate. |
| | PIP should remain < 30 cm $H_2O$ in infants and children. Higher PIPs should be avoided, if possible, but may be necessary in some patients with ↓CL. |
| | It is a misconception that PIP should be proportional to gestational age or weight. |
| | To recruit alveoli, appropriate PEEP is crucial. When high PIPs are used to open closed alveoli, the open alveoli may over-distend, resulting in volutrauma. |
| **Cautions** | ***In Pressure Ventilation, PIP and mPAW must often be decreased quickly when surfactant is administered.*** |
| | Rapidly changing (increasing) CL and FRC places the patient at high risk for lung over-distension and resultant air leaks. VT should be continuously monitored. |
| | It is critically important to understand the difference between ventilators that are PEEP-compensated and ones that are not (see caution below). |
| **Selecting Initial PIP** | PIP is set in pressure modes: |
| | 1. Adjust PIP to a target tidal volume range |
| | 2. Use the Pressure-Volume Loop: adjust PIP until there is little or no flattening of the loop |

**Caution**: Some ventilators (and some versions of the same ventilator) have a set Pressure Control (PIP) above the set PEEP, while in others the set Pressure Control is the "true" PIP (above baseline). Sometimes this is also referred to as **PEEP-compensated** or **not-PEEP-compensated**.

| Mean Airway Pressure (mPAW) | |
| --- | --- |
| **Normal Range** | 5-15 cm $H_2O$ |
| **Clinical Notes** | **mPAW** is often the most critical factor in determining optimal oxygenation as it correlates with lung volume. Generally, there is a linear rise in mean $PaO_2$ with ↑ mPAW until over-distension occurs, then a ↓ $PaO_2$ (and ↑ $PaCO_2$) occurs. <br><br> *Factors affecting mPAW (in probable order of magnitude):* PEEP, TI, PIP, $f$ (↓TE), VI, and pressure waveform (see diagram below) <br><br> **Approximation of mPAW:** <br> $$mPAW = \left[ \frac{(PIP \times TI)}{Cycle\ Time + (PEEP \times TE)} \right]$$ <br> Total Cycle Time <br><br> *Optimal level:* The lowest level in which gas exchange is most efficient and beyond which alveolar over-distension occurs |
| **Cautions** | In pressure ventilation, PIP and mPAW must often be decreased quickly when surfactant is administered <br><br> Rapidly changing (increasing) CL and FRC places the patient at high risk for lung over-distension and resultant air leaks (VILI) |

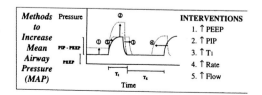

| Methods to Increase Mean Airway Pressure (MAP) | Pressure | INTERVENTIONS |
| --- | --- | --- |
| | | 1. ↑ PEEP |
| | | 2. ↑ PIP |
| | | 3. ↑ TI |
| | | 4. ↑ Rate |
| | | 5. ↑ Flow |

| Positive End Expiratory Pressure (PEEP) | |
|---|---|
| **Usual Range** | 4-7 cm $H_2O$ |
| **Clinical Notes** | PEEP is used to prevent airway/alveolar collapse and establish functional residual capacity (FRC). |
| **Cautions** | Setting PEEP is patient-specific. Focus on an optimal PEEP strategy versus specific PEEP levels<br><br>As the infant progresses, PEEP needs are likely to change. PEEP that is too low may result in poor oxygenation, surfactant deficiency, and ↑ risk of lung injury<br><br>PEEP that is too high may result in over-distension and may result in incomplete exhalation, ↑ PVR, ↓ CO (↓ venous return to heart)<br><br>Use caution to maintain PEEP when providing manual resuscitation |
| **Selecting Initial PEEP** (with example disease states - see Disease chapter for specific recommendations) | **Sub-Therapeutic PEEP: < 4 cm $H_2O$**<br><br>**Low PEEP:**   Overcome ET Tube resistance<br>4-5 cmH₂O   Prevent airway collapse<br><br>**Low-Mod PEEP:** Surfactant deficiency<br>5-7 cm $H_2O$   Air Leak<br><br>**High PEEP:**   Abdominal distension<br>8-10 cmH₂O   L-R Shunt |
| **Optimal PEEP** | 1. Use P-V loop (between lower and upper inflection points)<br>2. Incremental PEEP (increase PEEP, monitor change in VT with close watch of hemodynamics) |
| **Monitoring** | Increase in $PaO_2$<br>CXR: monitor under/over expansion<br>P-V Loop: shift of PIP down at same VT (remember VT should be set) |

## Frequency (*f*) or Rate

| | |
|---|---|
| **Usual Range** | 20-60 breaths/min |
| **Clinical Notes** | Used most commonly to adjust $PaCO_2$ and pH<br>General rule of thumb: ↓ CL requires ↑ *f*<br>The rate should be set in context of disease state, infant size and gestational age, clinical response.<br>Most clinicians allow for a ventilator rate that is less than the infant's drive (assuming a patient-triggered mode). Adequacy of rate can be assessed by physical assessment, pH, and $PaCO_2$. |
| **Cautions** | High rates = ↓ TE and may lead to air-trapping with inadvertent PEEP, and ↓ venous return and ↓ CO |

| Inspiratory Time (TI) | | | |
|---|---|---|---|
| **Usual Range** | LBW: 0.25 - 0.35 sec<br>Term: 0.3 - 0.4 sec | | |
| **Clinical Notes** | Select TI for patient comfort and synchronous breathing. Considerations include lung time constants, patient age, and breathing pattern. | | |

| $\downarrow$ CL | short TC (surfactant deficiency) | Use short TI ~0.3 sec |
|---|---|---|
| $\uparrow$ Raw | Long TC (BPD) | Use long TI ~0.5 sec |

TC = Time Constant

| **Cautions** | The longer the TI (especially > 1.0 sec), the greater the risk of barotrauma, adverse cardiac effects.<br>Longer TI = $\downarrow$ TE at same rate |
|---|---|

## STUDENT tip

Remember that neonates, infant, and young children have significantly higher respiratory rates. This will result in a much shorter Total Cycle Time (TCT = 60/$f$), which decreases inspiratory time and then available expiratory time

| Inspiratory Flow ($\dot{V}I$) | |
|---|---|
| **Normal Range** | LBW: 5-8 L/min<br>Term: 6-10 L/min |
| **Clinical Notes** | **Pressure Ventilation:** Flow is determined by patient characteristics<br><br>**Volume-Targeted Ventilation:** a pressure mode of ventilation (the name can be misleading). Tidal volume is set, and pressure is automatically titrated to deliver the targeted tidal volume. Flow should be sufficient to reach the necessary PIP.<br><br>**Volume Ventilation** (if able to set):<br>See Pediatric Ventilation (page 11-13) |
| **Cautions** | **Signs of insufficient flow:**<br>• Desired PIP not reached with mandatory breaths<br>• ↑ WOB (retractions, etc.)<br>• Pressure fluctuations on manometer around baseline PEEP setting<br>• Ventilator asynchrony |

Neonatal

Ventilation

| Flow Waveforms ($\dot{V}I$) | | |
|---|---|---|
| Decelerating Wave (descending ramp) | **Advantages** | Highest level of flow is at start of breath when patient flow demand is usually the greatest<br>May contribute to better patient-ventilator synchrony<br>Lower PIP (vs square)<br>Higher mPAW for equivalent PIP |
| | **Adverse Effects** | May result in ↓ venous return / CO (due to ↑ mPAW)<br>May result in ↓ expiratory time (vs square) |
| Sine Wave | **Advantages** | Smoother ↑ of pressure<br>More like normal respiratory pattern |
| | **Adverse Effects** | Lower mPAW |
| Square Wave (constant flow) | **Advantages** | Higher mPAW for equivalent PIP<br>Longer time at PIP may open atelectatic areas of lung and improve distribution of ventilation |
| | **Adverse Effects** | With high flow the ventilation may be applying higher pressures to normal airways and alveoli<br>Impedes venous return if longer Ti is used or I:E ratio is reversed |

*Much of this is theoretical with no sufficient evidence to back it.*

| Inspiratory:Expiratory Ratio (I:E Ratio) | |
|---|---|
| **Usual Range** | 1:1 to 1:3 |
| **Clinical Notes** | **I:E Ratio is usually not set directly.** Setting the RR and TI (or Flow Rate) determines the I:E Ratio.<br>PaCO₂ is seldom altered significantly by altering I:E Ratio. Altering PIP and PEEP is usually more effective. |
| **Cautions** | Inverse ratios carry a high risk of auto-PEEP and the potential for hyperinflation, barotrauma, ↓ CO, and cerebral injury |

*Although TE is not set, it is important for clinicians to understand its presence and ensure adequate passive exhalation time.*

| Expiratory Time (TE) | |
|---|---|
| **Normal Range** | 0.5 - 1.5 sec |
| **Clinical Notes** | **TE is usually not set**, but is the result of the rate and TI<br>$T_E = (60/f) - T_I$ |
| **Cautions** | Inverse ratios carry a high risk of auto-PEEP and the potential for hyperinflation, barotrauma, ↓ CO, and cerebral injury |

| Oxygen Percentage (O₂ %) |
|---|
| Fraction of Inspired Oxygen (FIO₂) -- decimal equivalent |

| | |
|---|---|
| **Possible Range** | 0.21 - 1.0 (21% - 100%) |
| **Clinical Notes** | It is very unusual to use more than minimum oxygen percentages in neonatal populations. The clinical consequences of moderate-to-high levels of oxygen are well documented. **The goal of care is to use the lowest amount of O₂ possible to meet minimum oxygenation goals.**<br><br>Clinicians should avoid, whenever possible, frequent changes in response to changing SpO₂ ("chasing the pulse ox") |
| **Cautions** | Hyperoxemia increases risk of Retinopathy of Prematurity (ROP) and Bronchopulmonary Dysplasia (BPD) |

| Leak Compensation | |
|---|---|
| **Overview** | An algorithm/setting on some neonatal ventilators that attempts to compensate for leakage (nares/mouth in noninvasive; ET tube in invasive), by calculating leakage and adjusting trigger sensitivity to allow for easier triggering without autocycling.<br><br>**The algorithm[1]:**<br>• Leakage flow is monitored by the ventilator (based on measured pressure and flow impedance) which is then subtracted from measured flow.<br>• The trigger sensitivity is adjusted automatically to maintain sensitivity without auto-cycling. |
| **Clinical Notes** | Noninvasive: neonatal interfaces usually loosely seal the nares (but not mouth), and in some cases even only use one nare.<br>Invasive: neonatal endotracheal tubes are usually cuffless which results in variable leaks (dependent on infant and tube size)<br>This can create a signficant issue with spontaneous ventilation (triggering and cycling).<br>If auto-triggering, the clinician could decrease trigger sensitivity (make it harder to trigger a breath), but the cost of this is trigger delay (it takes longer to reach the new, more difficult threshold)<br>There is variation in the leak compensation abilities of noninvasive and invasive ventilators. Clinicians need to be familiar with the ventilators used and be watching for possible synchrony issues.<br>In PSV with leak compensation, cycle off may be automatically set (see manufacturer literature) |

[1] Itagaki T, Chenell CT, Bennett DJ, Fisher DF, Kacmarek RM. Effects of Leak Compensation on Patient-Ventilator Synchrony During Premature/Neonatal Invasive and Noninvasive Ventilation: A Lung Model Study. Respiratory Care 2016

## Nasal CPAP

### Indications[1]

Note that this list is flexible. Many clinicians will trial CPAP for many situations, unless contraindicated.

| | |
|---|---|
| **Respiratory Distress** | ↑ RR (> 30% of normal)<br>Retractions (substernal, suprasternal)<br>Grunting<br>Nasal flaring<br>Pale or cyanotic skin color<br>Agitation |
| **Inadequate ABGs** | Inability to maintain $PaO_2$ > 50 mm Hg with $FIO_2$ ≤ 30% (assumes adequate $\dot{V}E$) |
| **Deteriorating CXR** | Presence of poorly expanded and/or infiltrated lung fields |
| **Specific Times** | RDS, Pulmonary edema<br>Atelectasis<br>Apnea of Prematurity<br>Recent extubation<br>Tracheal malacia |
| **Early Intervention** | With surfactant administration for VLBW infants<br>Immediately after delivery in preterm infants |
| **Weaning** | Commonly used to wean from invasive ventilation to a noninvasive CPAP - "step-down." |
| **Differentiate Between Cardiac and Pulmonary Cyanosis** | Give CPAP trial: |

| | Pulmonary | PPHN or CHD |
|---|---|---|
| $PaO_2$ (mmHg) | ↑ by > 20 | ↓ or no change |
| $PaCO_2$ (mmHg) | ↓ or no change | ↑ |

### Contraindications[1]

*When CPAP is contraindicated, it is because the infant requires immediate intubation.  Do not delay intubation when indicated.*

| Absolute | Diaphragmatic hernia (intubate immediately) |
|---|---|
| **Disease States** *(use with caution in these disease states)* | Cardiovascular instability<br>Choanal atresia<br>Cleft palate<br>Inadequate respiratory drive<br>TE fistula / Esophageal atresia |
| **Progressive Respiratory Failure** | Increasing apneas (frequency, duration) (frequency and severity, or with cyanosis)<br>Increasing $FIO_2$ > 60-70%<br>Increasing WOB (retractions, tachypnea, exhaustion, ↓ RR, gasping)<br>Worsening ABGs (respiratory acidosis) |

## Hazards

- Abdominal distention (may worsen with ↑ CPAP levels):  Place naso- or orogastric tube
- Existing cardiovascular impairment (may worsen with ↑ CPAP levels)
- $CO_2$ retention
- Overdistention and ↓ CL (may worsen with ↑ CPAP levels)
- ↑ risk of air leaks
- May ↑ PVR
- ↑ Intracranial Pressure (ICP)

[1]*These guidelines are largely summarized from:*
***AARC Expert Panel Reference-Based Guidelines***
*Application of continuous positive airway pressure to neonates via nasal prongs, or nasopharyngeal tube, or nasal mask*

## Noninvasive CPAP: Physiological Effects

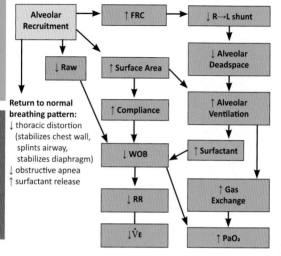

**Neonatal**

Alveolar Recruitment → ↑ FRC → ↓ R→L shunt → ↓ Alveolar Deadspace → ↑ Alveolar Ventilation

Alveolar Recruitment → ↓ Raw

Alveolar Recruitment → ↑ Surface Area → ↑ Compliance → ↓ WOB

↑ Alveolar Ventilation → ↑ Gas Exchange

**Ventilation**

**Return to normal breathing pattern:**
↓ thoracic distortion
  (stabilizes chest wall,
   splints airway,
   stabilizes diaphragm)
↓ obstructive apnea
↑ surfactant release

↑ Surfactant → ↓ WOB

↓ WOB → ↓ RR → ↓V̇E

↑ Gas Exchange → ↑ PaO₂

## CPAP Interfaces

| Method | Advantages | Disadvantages |
|---|---|---|
| **Nasal Prongs (N-CPAP) or Nasopharyngeal Prongs (NP-CPAP)** | May produce CPAP-like effect<br>Ease of application<br>Avoids complications of invasive intubation<br>Good accessibility to the patient<br>Mouth leak provides pressure release pop-off<br>Minimal cost | Irritating to skin and nasal septum<br>↑ WOB<br>Remove and clean every 2 hrs to reduce nasal irritation and skin breakdown<br>Mouth leak may result in loss of pressure<br>Crying causes pressure loss (and Room Air being inhaled—consider a chin strap) |
| **RAM Cannula** | Prongs are larger bore than conventional or high flow cannulas<br>Design allows for higher flow- and pressure-delivery without occluding nares<br>Prongs take up 60-80% of nares. Does not require a tight seal<br>Can provide noninvasive ventilation | May irritate nasal septum<br>During periods of crying, there may be a loss of pressure<br>May not note displacement until SpO₂ drops<br>When used as CPAP (no expiratory limb) has a high resistance to flow (delivered CPAP is ~2-3 cm H₂O less than set value). |
| **Endotracheal Tube CPAP** | Low gas flows can be used<br>High CPAP pressures obtained with low flows<br>Can easily switch to ventilator mode<br>Access to the infant is greatest<br>Leaks are more easily managed | Invasive, acute airway trauma and/or infection<br>Same concerns as ET Tubes in general<br>Tracheal stenosis, scarring, irritation possible<br>↑ Upper airway resistance<br>↑ WOB<br>Eliminates infant's ability to grunt |

| Method | Advantages | Disadvantages |
|--------|-----------|---------------|
| **Face Mask** (used during resuscitation, manually held in place) | Simple, easy to use<br>Less WOB than prongs | Temporary use during distress<br>Severe gastric distention (Place NG/OG)<br>Pressure necrosis<br>Cerebral hemorrhage<br>Gastric rupture<br>Hypercapnia due to increased deadspace |
| **Nasal Masks** | Less deadspace than face mask<br>Good accessibility to patient | During periods of crying, may lose pressure<br>Irritation/breakdown to bridge of nose* |

*Some facilities will alternate between nasal prongs and nasal masks in order to maintain skin integrity.

## Types of Nasal CPAP Produced

| How CPAP is delivered | Described Modes (letter correlate with mode descriptions that follow) |
|---|---|
| **Continuous Flow** delivers a relatively variable pressure (CPAP delivered may be inconsistent) | Bubble CPAP (A) |
| **Variable Flow** delivers a fairly stable pressure by altering flow (delivers more flow during inspiration, less flow during exhalation) | Variable Flow (B) |

### Clinical Note:

Some clinicians utilize a High Flow Nasal Cannula (HFNC) for its inadvertent PEEP (higher flows may cause expiratory resistance). It is important to understand the potential expiratory resistance that can occur. A HFNC is not a CPAP-device, and does not cause expiratory resistance when flows are set correctly. CPAP-devices should be used when CPAP is required.

| Bubble Nasal CPAP (B-NCPAP) | A |
|---|---|
| **How it Works** | Provides a set CPAP (the distal end of expiratory tubing is placed below the water seal surface), releasing pressure via bubbles. Provides some oscillation on the inside of the airways (versus externally such as through chest physiotherapy) which have been theorized to improve interregional gas mixing and alveolar recruitment. |
| **Classification** | Constant-flow |
| **Use Notes** | Once set-up, a leak test should be performed (bubbling will be noted)<br>Flow rate is usually set at 6-8 L/min (4-15 L/min is allowable range)<br>Set CPAP level[1]. It is recommended that numbers on the (equipment's) column are used as a rough starting point, then verify delivered pressure using a pressure manometer positioned at the nasal prongs.<br>**Condensation in the expiratory limb may lead to higher pressures than intended being delivered.** Ensure optimal humidity, but ensure condensate is emptied frequently from the limb. |

[1] May underestimate actual delivered pressures.

## Variable-Flow N-CPAP
**Hamilton Medical** *Arabella,*
**Care Fusion** *Infant Flow (NCPAP)*

| | |
|---|---|
| **How it Works** | Delivered flow is varied.  Flow towards the patient increases slightly during inspiration and decreases slightly during exhalation (results in a more constant pressure delivery). |
| | This uses the construct of Bernoulli, Coanda, and Venturi principles. |
| **Classification** | Variable-Flow, Constant-Pressure |
| **Use Notes** | Arabella has pressure monitor at the proximal side |

## ■ CPAP: Initiation and Management

The following are general guidelines.

**Initiate** CPAP at 5-6 cmH₂O

**Adjust** CPAP for continued hypoxemia (PaO₂ < 50 mm Hg):
1. Increase CPAP in 1 cmH₂O intervals to a total CPAP of 8 initially (higher may be needed).
2. Increase O₂% in increments of 5-10%.
   Adjust O₂ to keep PaO₂ > 50 mm Hg; SpO₂ ~90-95%.
3. Full support ventilation if determined to be failing CPAP

### Monitoring Patients on CPAP

- Abnominal distention and bowel sounds
- Skin color and integrity
- ABGs or CBGs with SpO₂
- Chest X-Ray (CXR)
- Vital Signs (HR, RR, BP, temperature)
- WOB (RR, pattern, grunting, retractions)
- Ensure proper interface - a tight seal is not usually needed
- Proper Sizing: Nasal prongs should fill nares, but not cause any blanching (which will lead to skin/tissue breakdown)
- CPAP: pressure, pop-off, leaks
- Gas temperature, humidity

### Hazards in CPAP

Air leaks
Aspiration
Feeding intolerance
Gastric distention/rupture
Hypothermia
Increased ICP (IVH)
Infection (if ET Tube)
Muscle fatigue
Pneumothorax/PIE

Pulmonary edema
Recurrent apnea
Respiratory failure
Tube/prong obstruction,
   dislodgement, irritation,
Nasal necrosis
Under- or over-hydration
Low- or high-device temp.

## Indications of CPAP Success (and suggested actions)

| | |
|---|---|
| **Inadequate CPAP (↓)**<br><br>*Increase CPAP in increments* | Continued respiratory distress<br>SpO₂ may not change, or gradually worsen<br>RR: no change or worsens<br>CXR: no change or worsens |
| **Adequate CPAP** | ↑ PaO₂ (SpO₂)<br>RR towards normal<br>↓ WOB<br>CXR: improved aeration |
| **Optimal CPAP** | To determine, look for highest SpO₂ without a significant change in pH/PaCO₂ or cardio-vascular status |
| **Excessive CPAP (↑)**<br><br>*Decrease CPAP immediately* | Gastric distention<br>Vomiting<br>↓ Cardiac Output (CV instability) |

**Indications of CPAP Failure (any one of the following):**
- $PaO_2$ < 50 mm Hg or $SpO_2$ < 85% on $O_2$% > 60%
- Hypercapnia
- pH < 7.20 (respiratory)
- Apnea and bradycardia
- Change in level of consciousness (lethargy, unresponsiveness)
- Respiratory distress

**Selected Causes of CPAP Failure:**
- Apneas (frequent and/or causing bradycardia)
- Atelectasis persisting (ineffective CPAP)
- Intraventricular hemorrhage (IVH)
- Muscle fatigue (nutrition, prematurity)
- Metabolic acidosis
- Pulmonary edema

## ■ CPAP: Weaning

**When to Wean:**
- ABGs improving (SpO₂ ≥ 95% or PaO₂ ≥ 70 mm Hg)
- CXR improving (increased aeration/expansion)
- No apneas
- Any respiratory distress has resolved
- Vital signs stable

**Weaning Process**
1. ↓ FiO₂ aggressively before weaning CPAP
2. ↓ CPAP in increments of 1-2 cm H₂O
3. Remove CPAP when O₂% = 21-25% on CPAP +5 cm H₂O with no respiratory distress

**Clinical Notes**
- Maintain SpO₂ 90 - 95%, PaO₂ 50 - 70 mm Hg, PaCO₂ < 55 mm Hg, and pH > 7.25
- Incremental changes may be made as often as every 2 hours
- Obtain CXR to assess for adequate lung inflation
- Stop wean if PaO₂ < 50 mm Hg or retractions increase

**Monitor closely after removal.** Watch for apneas, bradycardia, tachypnea, retractions

**See Also: Supplemental Oxygen for details on low-flow and high-flow oxygen delivery (pages 5-17, 12-27))**

## ■ Noninvasive Positive Pressure Ventilation (NIPPV)

Maintains a higher mPAW than N-CPAP, allowing for better recruitment, ↑ FRC, resulting in improved oxygenation. Providing a second level of pressure allows for some gas exchange and further prevents airway collapse.

### Goals

- Assist weak or ineffective spontaneous breathing
- Avoid endotrauma (airway/lung injury during and sometimes after being intubated and on an invasive ventilator)
- Act as a bridge for premature neonates who would otherwise fail N-CPAP or remain intubated

### Interface

Most common:  short nasal prongs (same as used for N-CPAP)
Less common:  nasopharyngeal tube which is inserted 2-3 cm into a single nare, leaving the other nare as an additional pressure-relief valve.

### Modes include:

| Noninvasive Positive Pressure Ventilation (NIPPV) |
| --- |
| N-IMV (C) |
| NIV-NAVA (see invasive modes for details) |
| SiPAP (D) |
| N-HFV (E) |

| Nasal Intermittent Mandatory Ventilation (N-IMV, NIPPV) | C |
|---|---|

| How it Works | Used with conventional ventilation with short prongs (or nasopharyngeal ET Tube) to provide mandatory breaths<br>Available as:<br>• Synchronized (SNIPPV) - not available in U.S.<br>• Unsynchronized (NIPPV) |
|---|---|
| Classification | Time-triggered, Pressure-limited, Time-cycled |
| Parameters | • Inspiratory Pressure<br>• Rate<br>• Inspiratory Time<br>• Positive End Expiratory Pressure (PEEP)<br>• Oxygen Percentage ($O_2$%, $FIO_2$) |
| Complications | • Gastric insufflation/perforation<br>• Risk for lung injury still exists |
| Clinical Notes | • Pressure Support can not be used with the spontaneous breaths in this mode (the leak makes it difficult to flow cycle breaths)<br>• Neonates can not trigger in IMV. |

**Suggested Initial Settings[1]**

| IP | 2-4 $cmH_2O$ > Prior Vent PIP or 16-20 cm $H_2O$<br>Do not exceed 25 cm $H_2O$ |
|---|---|
| PEEP | Same as Vent PEEP ~4-6 cm $H_2O$ |
| f | 20-40 breaths/min (at least 50% of total RR if Synchronized - where available) |
| TI | 0.30-0.4 sec ($\dot{V}I$ 8-10 L/min) |

[1] Adapted from Bhandari, J Perinatology, 2010, 30:505-512

| | |
|---|---|
| **How it Works** | CPAP generator that allows the infant to breathe spontaneously at 2 separate CPAP levels (in BiPhasic mode). Additional flow is diverted to the infant during the sigh interval, increasing inspiratory pressure (acting as a recruitment tool) |
| **Classification** | CPAP: Variable-flow, Variable-pressure<br>Assist: Time-triggered, Pressure-limited |
| **Use Notes** | Interface via nasal mask or nasal prongs<br>Pressure is monitored at interface<br>Pressure levels are set by flow<br>N-CPAP is single level<br>BiPhasic includes NCPAP (low) +<br>               Phigh (the sigh interval)<br>PIPs generated are usually ~9-11 cm $H_2O$ |

**Typical Initial Settings**

| NCPAP (Pressure Low) | 8 L/min (produces ~ 5 cm $H_2O$ pressure at low level) |
|---|---|
| Pressure High | 3 L/min above low (11 L/min) (2-4 cm $H_2O$ above low) |
| Time High | minimum of 0.4-1.0 sec |
| Rate | This is frequency of sigh (when pressure high is applied) 10-20 breaths/min |

*Pressure High* should be thought of as OVER *Pressure Low* - this is the delta P (change in pressure) which determines the amount of support the patient is receiving.

| Nasal High Frequency Ventilation (N-HFV) | E |
|---|---|
| **How it Works** | Noninvasive ventilation mode that applies an oscillatory (back and forth) pressure waveform to the airways via either short prongs or naso-pharyngeal nasal ET tube.<br><br>Inspiration and exhalation are usually active<br>Gas flows are sinusoidal |
| **Classification** | Usually:<br>Time-cycled, Pressure-limited<br>(with oscillations) |
| **Benefits** | This mode may better facilitate $CO_2$ removal compared to N-CPAP<br>This mode may eliminate the need for synchronization |
| **Use Notes** | Though theoretically useful, N-HFV requires more evidence-based support.<br><br>There are several ventilators equipped to handle N-HFV, including notably Percussionaire Intrapulmonary Percussive Ventilation (IPV) - including the VDR - which uses a phasitron to deliver bursts of gas. |

# ◼ Conventional Ventilation: Modes
**Pressure vs. Volume Ventilation**

> **True volume ventilation**, with large volumes injected into the circuit, can only be used in large patients with cuffed ET tubes, and so is rarely used in babies. It is theoretically possible with the placement of a proximal flow sensor[1].
>
> **Volume-targeted ventilation** (this is a <u>pressure-control</u> mode that attempts to deliver a set tidal volume) has been shown to decrease mortality, morbidity, and ventilator days compared to pressure-control ventilation without volume targeting[2,3].

## Neonatal Modes
*In-depth information for each mode is found on the following pages*

| Pressure Ventilation | Volume Ventilation<br>*not typically used in NICU*<br>*(presented here for continuity)* |
|---|---|
| P-SIMV (F) | V-SIMV  (SEE page 11-23) |
| PC-A/C (G) | VC-A/C  (SEE page 11-25) |
| PS (H) | *Volume-targeted modes of ven-tilation are pressure ventilation (the pressure varies to target a set tidal volume)* |
| **Volume-Targeted Ventilation** | |
| PRVC (I) | |
| VG (J) | |
| **Other** | |
| NAVA (K) | |
| **High Frequency** | |
| HFOV (L) | HFJV (M) |

[1] Goldsmith, J, Karotkin E, Suresh G, Keszler M.  Assisted Ventilation of the Neonate. Saunders; 2016:197

[2] Peng, W, Zhu H, Shi H, Liu E.  Volume-targeted ventilation is more suitable than pressure-limited ventilation for preterm infants: A systematic review and meta-analysis. Archives of Disease in Childhood.  Fetal and Neonatal Edition 2014;99(2):158-165.

[3] Wheeler, K, Klingenberg, C, Morley, C, Davis, P.  Volume-targeted versus pressure-limited ventilation for preterm infants: A systematic review and meta-analysis. Neonatology.  2011;100(3):219-227.

## Pressure-Synchronized Intermittent Mandatory Ventilation    F
(P-SIMV)

| Summary | A combination of spontaneous and mandatory ventilation |
|---|---|
| | • The ventilator will deliver a set number of mandatory (controlled) breaths per minute |
| | • These mandatory breaths will be at a preset PIP and $T_i$ |
| | • The patient may breathe spontaneously in between the mandatory ventilator breaths from the baseline pressure. The breaths must be supported with pressure support |
| | • If the patient begins to inspire just prior to the time triggered mandatory (control) breath, a full machine-assisted breath will be delivered |
| | **It is common now to use a hybrid of this mode with a volume target** |

**\*\*Caution**: Some ventilators (and some versions of the same ventilator) have a set Pressure Control (PIP) above the set PEEP, while in others the set Pressure Control is the "true" PIP (above baseline). Sometimes this is also referred to as **PEEP-compensated** or **not-PEEP-compensated**.

| | Classified By: | | |
|---|---|---|---|
| Breath Type | Trigger | Limit | Cycle |
| **Mandatory** *(Controlled)* | MT *(Time)* | ML *(Press)* | MC *(Time)* |
| **Assisted** | PT *(Press or $\dot{V}$)* | ML *(Press)* | MC *(Time)* |
| **Spontaneous** | PT *(Press or $\dot{V}$)* | PL *(Press)* | PC *(Press or $\dot{V}$)* |

MT = Machine-triggered     PT = Patient-triggered
ML = Machine-limited        PL = Patient-limited
MC = Machine-cycled         PC = Patient-cycled

# P-SIMV

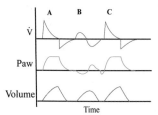

Breath A is controlled and time-triggered
Breath B is a spontaneous breath (no pressure support)
Breath C is synchronized and assisted
Breaths A and C are full machine pressure breaths

**Advantages**:
- Synchronization of spontaneous and machine breaths
- Delivers volume early in the breath, which may improve gas
  distribution

**Disadvantages and Risks**:
- No guaranteed $V_T$. (Set Low $V_T$ and $\dot{V}_E$ alarms carefully)
- Excessive patient WOB if the sensitivity is not set correctly
- Increased patient-ventilator asynchrony compared to continuous
  mandatory support modes

**Clinical Notes**
- May be well-suited for infants when apnea is primary indication
- If $f$ < 30 in low birthweight infant, extubate
- Inspiratory Pressure is usually set by a $V_T$ range, and then should
  be monitored closely as lung mechanics change
- Spontaneous breaths must be supported with pressure sup-
  port (SIMV without PS is contraindicated in infants due to the
  increased work of breathing of unsupported intubated breaths)

## Pressure Control / Assist-Control    G
(PC/AC or P-A/C or P/C-A/C)

| Summary | A combination of assisted and/or controlled (mandatory) ventilation |
|---------|------------------|
| | • All breaths are delivered at a preset PIP and T$_I$ |
| | • In between the controlled breaths a patient can trigger a full machine (assisted) breath at the same parameters as the controlled breath (i.e., PIP and T$_I$) |
| | **It is common now to use a hybrid of this mode with a volume target** |

**\*\*Caution**: Some ventilators (and some versions of the same ventilator) set Pressure Control (PIP) relative to the set PEEP, while in others the set Pressure Control is the "true" PIP (above baseline). Sometimes this is also referred to as **PEEP-compensated** or **not-PEEP-compensated**.

#### Other Names for Pressure-Assist/Control

Pressure Control
Pressure Assist Mechanical Ventilation

| Other Names for Assist | Other Names for Control |
|------------------------|-------------------------|
| Pressure Assist (PA) | Control Mode |
| Pressure Control Ventilation (PCV) | Controlled Mechanical Ventilation (CMV) |
| Assisted Ventilation (AV) | Pressure Control Ventilation (PCV) |
| Assisted Mechanical Ventilation (AMV) | |

| | Classified By: | | |
|------------|------------|------------|------------|
| **Breath Type** | **Trigger** | **Limit** | **Cycle** |
| **Mandatory** *(Controlled)* | MT *(Time)* | ML *(Press)* | MC *(Time)* |
| **Assisted** | PT *(Press or V̇)* | ML *(Press)* | MC *(Time)* |

MT = Machine-triggered    PT = Patient-triggered
ML = Machine-limited    PL = Patient-limited
MC = Machine-cycled    PC = Patient-cycled

## P-ACV

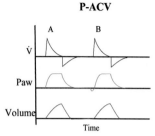

$\dot{V}$

Paw

Volume

Time

Breath A is controlled and time-triggered
Breath B is assisted and patient-triggered
Each breath is a full machine pressure breath

**Advantages:**
- Minimal patient WOB (if parameters are properly adjusted)
- Allows patient control of rate and $\dot{V}_E$
- Variable $\dot{V}_I$ may be more comfortable for patients
- Delivers volume early in the breath (decelerating flow) which may improve gas distribution

**Disadvantages and Risks:**
- No guaranteed $V_T$ (as in volume ventilation)
- Low exhaled $V_T$ and $\dot{V}_E$ alarms must be set properly
- May cause or worsen auto-PEEP (dynamic hyperinflation)

**Clinical Notes**
- The set rate (*f*) can be thought of as a back-up, or minimum, rate. It should be set just below the spontaneous rate (usually 30-40 breaths/min). Rationale: a rate set too slow may result in variation in minute ventilation and $O_2$ during neonatal apneas; a rate set too high results in ventilator triggering a breath before the infant has a chance to.
- Wean: Lower Inspiratory Pressure (IP). This allows the infant to assume more WOB. It is not advisable to lower the rate.

## Pressure Support Ventilation
(PSV)                                                       H

**Summary**

Spontaneous ventilation with all of the patient's spontaneous breaths supported or augmented by the ventilator (a set pressure is added to each spontaneous breath). It differs from P/C-A/C in that breaths are FLOW cycled, not TIME cycled.

In neonatal populations, PSV should always be used with SIMV (see SIMV, page 4-36) - it is critical to have a back-up rate.

In pediatric populations, PSV is often used as a weaning mode. Careful attention must be paid to setting acceptable back-up mode parameters (when applicable), as well as apnea time alarm.

# PSV

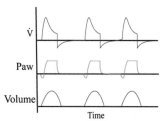

$\dot{V}$

Paw

Volume

Time

**Clinical Notes:**

There are specific challenges in using PSV with the infant population. Flow cycling works best with a sealed airway (ET tube with cuff inflated), but most infants have a cuffless ET tube with variance in leak sizes.

Some ventilators now compensate for this through leak compensation (i.e. leak-adapted pressure support in Drager Ventilators). The cycle off is set at 15% in these leak-compensating ventilators.

Breaths are flow-cycled: as the flow of the breath naturally slows (to a set % of peak expiratory flow), the ventilator allows the patient to transition into exhalation)

Switching from A/C modes to PSV usually ↓ mPAW (due to the tendency for TI to be smaller when pt-determine through flow cycling). It is important to compensate for this loss of mPAW with PEEP.

Tidal volume is dependent upon lung compliance and resistance, drive to breathe, and amount of pressure support.

Consider setting PS level at 30-50% of difference between PIP and PEEP

PS levels < 10 cm $H_2O$ (above PEEP) may be used if utilizing solely to overcome high resistance of ET Tube

It is critical to ensure a minimum mandatory backup rate in case of apnea

## Pressure-Regulated Volume Control
(PRVC)

| Summary | This is, at its foundation, a pressure controlled mode, but adds a target tidal volume, so that the inspiratory pressure changes breath-by-breath up to a set point in order to maintain a stable VT |
|---|---|

**Ventilator Specific**: PRVC-Maquet Servo I; Servo 300/300A **Viasys Avea and Viasys Vela

**Other Names:**  Variable Pressure Control (VPC),
Volume Control Plus (VCP), VC+)
**Refer to the manufacturer's manual (algorithms slightly different)

|  | Classified By: | | |
|---|---|---|---|
| **Breath Type** | **Trigger** | **Limit** | **Cycle** |
| **Mandatory** | MT *(Time)* | ML *(Press or Vol)* | MC *(Time)* |
| **Assisted** | PT *(Press or $\dot{V}$)* | ML *(Press or Vol)* | MC *(Time)* |

**How it works:**

- For the first breath, the ventilator gives a volume breath with a pause (plateau)
- The second breath will be a pressure breath at that plateau pressure from the previous breath
- The ventilator will then titrate the inspiratory pressure by no more than 3 $cmH_2O$ from one breath to the next in order to try to meet the target $V_T$
- As a safety, the maximum available pressure level is 5 $cmH_2O$ below the preset upper pressure alarm (alarm will sound at this point and the breath will switch into exhalation, meaning the set $V_T$ will not be fully delivered - the ventilator will only deliver the amount of volume that it can before hitting that upper limit)
- The minimum inspiratory pressure limit is the baseline setting (PEEP)
- The patient will receive a minimum number of time-triggered mandatory breaths per minute (as in PC-A/C)
- PRVC can be combined with SIMV (PRVC-SIMV) so that mandatory breaths are PRVC breaths, and spontaneous are PSV breaths

# PRVC

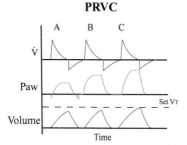

As the breaths advance from A to C, the pressure is automatically increased to achieve the set V$_T$.

**Advantages**:
- Guaranteed V$_T$ and $\dot{V}_E$
- Patient can breathe above the set $f$
- Allows patient control of RR and $\dot{V}_E$
- Variable $\dot{V}_I$ (decelerating) to meet patient demand and improve gas distribution

**Disadvantages and Risks**:
- **Upper pressure limit (alarm) must be set appropriately**
- Excessive patient work of breathing if sensitivity is not set correctly
- May cause or worsen auto-PEEP
- Patients who assist the ventilator by taking larger V$_T$ will cause the inspiratory pressure to drop (as the ventilator drops it in increments of 3's to try to get to goal V$_T$). If the patient then tires, the ventilator could be delivering as low as the PEEP level at a time when the patient most needs the support. A PIP dropping to PEEP level is a warning of this likelihood.

> **Adaptive Pressure Ventilation (APV)** is similar to PRVC with slight variation in the delivery algorithm and with high pressure limiting. See manufacturer's literature for exact details. Initiation, management, and troubleshooting are otherwise the same as with PRVC.

## Volume Guarantee

(VG)

**J**

| Summary | • **VOLUME TARGETED:** Uses a targeted (clinician-set) tidal volume - this is a minimum delivered tidal volume.<br>• Pressure automatically titrates in small increments to deliver preset VT<br>• Infants can breathe over the targeted tidal volume |

**Ventilation**

| | Classified By: | | |
|---|---|---|---|
| **Breath Type** | **Trigger** | **Limit** | **Cycle** |
| **Mandatory** *(Controlled)* | MT *(Time)* | PL *(Pressure)* | MC *(Time)* |

MT = Machine-triggered    PT = Patient-triggered
ML = Machine-limited       PL = Patient-limited
MC = Machine-cycled        PC = Patient-cycled

**How it Works**

1. Clinician sets a targeted tidal volume
2. A pressure breath is delivered: PEEP + 5 cm $H_2O$
3. Compliance is calculated
4. The next breath is delivered at 75% of the calculated pressure (CL)
5. The following breaths will titrate by up to 3 cm $H_2O$ to achieve the targeted tidal volume.

**Hazards**

If infant is crying or otherwise breathing hard, the ventilator will allow larger breaths to be taken, but will provide little to no support (no pressure assistance). This may result in fatigue.

## ■ Conventional Ventilation: Management

### Initiating Neonatal Invasive Ventilation
*See Parameters for guidelines on initiating ventilation*

*There are no rules or definitive guidelines for ventilation, only suggestions. All settings are variable and must be modified based upon the disease state, ventilation type, gestational age, postnatal age, and weight.*

*The goal should be to carefully support oxygen and ventilation needs while avoiding complications, particularly any harm.*

**Summary Overview of Initial Settings:**

| Parameter | Neonatal Setting |
|---|---|
| (Mode) | Volume-Targeted modes |
| $V_T$ | 4-6 mL/kg |
| PIP (Inspiratory Pressure) | 15-20 cm $H_2O$ |
| PEEP | 4-7 cm $H_2O$ |
| $T_i$ | 0.3 - 0.4 sec |
| $\dot{V}_i$ | 6-10 L/min |
| $FIO_2$ | As minimal as possible to maintain $SpO_2$ goal range |

> **See Specific Diseases/Disorders in Chapter 3 for Specific Recommendations, when available.**

# Oxygenation

In general, oxygenation goals are very conservative with neonates.

| Improving Oxygenation: PaO₂ (SaO₂, SpO₂) | |
|---|---|
| Goal | To maintain adequate $O_2$ delivery to the tissues while ventilating with the lowest possible $FiO_2$ and pressures. |
| Methods: Details following pages | ↑ FiO₂: Immediate but temporary measure for increasing the $O_2$ gradient |
| | Optimize mPAW: $V_T$, PIP, PEEP, $T_I$, $\dot{V}I$, $\dot{V}I$ waveform. This has a greater effect on V/Q matching and is often a key to improving and support oxygenation. |
| | Adequate $O_2$ delivery to tissues is dependent on $FiO_2$, CO, and $CaO_2$. |

## Quick Estimates of Oxygenation Status:

**P/F ratio** = $PaO_2 / F_IO_2$
- $PaO_2$ is the amount of oxygen in the arteries
- $FIO_2$ is the amount of oxygen in the alveoli (roughly, of course)
- The ratio estimates how well oxygen is getting from alveoli to the arteries.
- Normal is approximately 500

**Oxygen Index (OI)** = $\dfrac{F_IO_2 \times Paw \times 100}{PaO_2}$        $F_IO_2$ is a decimal!

OI again estimates the amount of oxygen that goes from alveoli to blood, but takes into account mean airway pressure, which we know is greatly impacted by factors like PEEP. Thus, the OI can be considered a more powerful estimate of oxygenation.

# Methods for Improving Oxygenation

Concept:  Increasing $FIO_2$ is a temporary measure, but has severe consequences for neonates.  Optimizing mPAW is critical.

1. Increase $FIO_2$ ($\uparrow O_2$ tension/gradient)
2. Optimize mPAW by PEEP
   (eliminate auto-PEEP, $\uparrow$ FRC, $\downarrow$ shunting)
3. Optimize mPAW other than by PEEP ($\uparrow$ FRC)
4. Position patient (optimize V/Q matching)

| 1. $F_IO_2$ | |
|---|---|
| Goal | Use the minimum amount of supplemental oxygen necessary to maintain <u>adequate</u> oxygenation (not necessarily normal oxygenation) |
| Principle | This is a major determinant of oxygenation, increasing the $P(A-a)O_2$ gradient, which usually results in a greater $PaO_2$. |
| Clinical Notes | Increase $FIO_2$ cautiously.  High $FIO_2$ over time may lead to oxygen toxicity, so the overall goal is to maintain as low as clinically possible. It is often preferred to optimize mPAW versus chasing the patient's $SpO_2$ using $FIO_2$. |

| 2. PEEP | |
|---|---|
| Goal | OPTIMAL PEEP which:<br>↑ $PaO_2$ – ↓ shunt effect, ↑ FRC, and ↑ CL, allowing for the reduction of $FiO_2$ and its complications.<br>↓ **WOB** – Unload the inspiratory muscles |
| Principle | Determinant of oxygenation by affecting Paw. |
| Clinical Notes | Maintains pressures above ambient pressure during the expiratory phase to prevent collapse of smaller airways and unstable alveoli. |
| Contrain-dications | **Absolute**:<br>Tension Pneumothorax<br>Untreated Pneumothorax (significant in size)<br><br>**Relative**:<br>• Barotrauma<br>• Bronchopulmonary fistula<br>• Pre-existing hyperinflation<br>• Hypovolemia<br>• Recent lung surgery<br>• Unilateral lung disorders |

**Beneficial Effects of Appropriate PEEP**

↑ $\overline{Paw}$ ↑ CL ↑ $PaO_2$ (for a given $FiO_2$) ↓ WOB

↑ V/Q (the stabilization of collapsing alveoli resulting in improved gas distribution and ↓ R-L shunting).

↑ FRC (which may include recruitment of collapsed alveoli)

↓ Lung injury (minimizes shear forces)

PEEP may be beneficial in patients with CHF by ↓ preload and afterload.

**Potential Adverse Effects of Inappropriate PEEP**

Alveolar over-distension (volutrauma – which is proportional to lung disease, over-distension, and pressure), ↑ WOB, ↑ $V_D/V_T$.

Cardiovascualr effects are dependent on PEEP level, $C_{LT}$, and cardiovascular status. The greatest effect (↓ venous return and ↓ cardiac output) is when CL is high, chest wall compliance is low, and cardiovascualr reserve is low.

*Renal function* - May ↓ renal and portal blood flow, hence ↓ UO.

*ICP* - When PEEP decreases venous return, ICP may ↑. Usually clinically insignificant unless ICP is already elevated. Head elevation may offset PEEP effect.

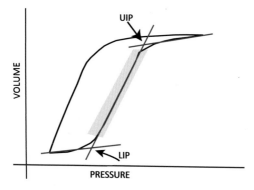

### Understanding the P-V Loop and PEEP:

1. The steep part of the curve represents rapid increases in Volume with small pressure changes, implying best compliance as the lungs accept volume easily.

2. The flattened sections represent areas where it takes greater pressures to move small volumes of air (the cost of ventilation, and the risk of lung damage, is high):

   **Lower**: Lower flattened section suggests areas of the lungs that are closing and opening, which results in atelectrauma. These are separated in the above diagram by the Lower Inflection Point (LIP).

   **Upper**: Upper flattened section ("duckbill"), when present, suggests over-distension, which can lead to barotrauma (damage caused by excessive pressure).  PEEP should always be set below the Upper Inflection Point (UIP).

3. The slope of the curve provides information about lung compliance.  Less steep curves suggest poor compliance (it always takes a fair amount of pressure to deliver a volume)

4. Ideally this curve is captured with no patient contribution, meaning it is most accurate when a patient is given a single-dose of a paralytic. Note that the LIP in particular is not always discernible.

| 3. Mean Airway Pressure ($\overline{P}aw$ or MAWP or MAP or mPAW) | |
|---|---|
| **Goal** | Achieve adequate oxygenation with the lowest possible pressures and $F_IO_2$ without impairing CV function or injuring the lungs |
| **Principle** | Paw is an important determinant of oxygenation $PaO_2 \sim \overline{P}aw$ (until overdistension occurs) |
| **Indication** | $\uparrow$ Paw is indicated for patients with risk of—or presence of — $\downarrow$ lung volumes and refractory hypoxemia (does not respond to increasing the $F_IO_2$) Refractory Hypoxemia = $PaO_2 < 60$ mmHg on $F_IO_2 > 0.6$ |

**Primary Factors Affecting $\overline{P}aw$** (in probable order of influence)

- PEEP
- PIP
- $T_I$
- $f (\downarrow T_E)$
- $\dot{V}_I$
- $\dot{V}_I$ waveform

Clinical Note: Limit $T_I$ to the maximum that does not cause auto-PEEP.
If auto-PEEP present:     In Volume: auto-PEEP $\rightarrow \uparrow$Palv ($V_T$ constant)
                                    In Pressure: auto-PEEP $\rightarrow \downarrow V_T$ (Palv constant)

**Potential Risks of** $\uparrow \overline{P}aw$ = barotrauma, $\downarrow$ CO

**Measurement Of $\overline{P}aw$**

| Automatically calculated by ventilator | Manually calculated |
|---|---|
| Note: this value usually doesn't include any auto-PEEP | $\overline{P}aw = (PIP - PEEP) \times (T_I / T_{total}) + PEEP$ (figuring a constant flow, volume breath and PEEP includes auto-PEEP) |

| 4. Patient Positioning | |
|---|---|
| **Goal** | Improve V/Q and FRC by placing patient in various positions - usually either lateral (right side down or left side down) or by proning patient (stomach down) |
| **Principle** | This may assist with oxygenation by aligning perfusion (blood will go wherever gravity takes it — down) WITH ventilation (placing the better lung regions where the best perfusion is). The goal is to align good lung with good perfusion, as much as possible.<br><br>BLU GLD (remember it as: Blue Gold) =<br>               Bad Lung UP, Good Lung DOWN<br>(Except with pulm hemorrhage, lung abscess) |
| **Contrain-dication** | **Absolute**:<br>Spinal cord instability<br>**Relative**:<br>Thoracic/Abdominal surgeries (recent)<br>Hemodynamic/Cardiovascular instability |
| **Clinical Notes** | • Careful monitoring of ventilator parameters and patient deterioration, complications, line/tube placement, etc., is essential during and directly following repositioning<br>• Improvement is most likely within 30 minutes |

**Neonatal**

**Ventilation**

**Procedure**:
- Ensure team members are in place (including 1 person in charge of monitoring secure airway/vent circuit)
- Disconnect all leads/lines as necessary
- Gently place pt. on side
- Verify status of pt./equipment/lines
- Place patient in prone position
- Turn patient's head towards the ventilator
- Reattach and verify all leads/lines - ensure that the ET tube/head are not compressed
- Do a complete ventilator-patient check, including breath sounds
- Again verify vital signs and hemodynamic status

## Ventilation

| Improving Ventilation: PaCO$_2$ (and pH) | |
|---|---|
| Goal | Maintain adequate CO$_2$ elimination while protecting the lungs from injury. |
| Principle | Adequacy of ventilation is mostly determined by minute ventilation, and assessed by PaCO$_2$/pH (Several therapeutic strategies exist, including lung protection) |
| | PaCO$_2$ and resultant pH are impacted by total ventilation, deadspace, and CO$_2$ production. They are changed by altering minute ventilaton, deadspace and/or CO$_2$ production. Note that deadspace is not often used therapeutically anymore. |
| Methods | **Manipulating ventilation occurs in two ways:** |
| | 1. **Tidal Volume ($\Delta P$ in pressure control modes)** Typically set to a range based upon height (ideal body weight). There is usually wiggle room within that range for minor adjustments, but ultimately is a "set and forget" parameter. |
| | 2. **Ventilator Rate ($f$)** More typically manipulated to alter minute ventilation in either volume or pressure control modes. Changing $f$ also changes I:E ratio, so care must be taken to ensure adequate exhalation time. |
| | Manipulating these parameters is dependent on mode, patient's spontaneous (total) rate, spontaneous tidal volume in some modes, inspiratory time, disease process, etc. |
| | **Independent of disease processes:** |
| | • ↑ VT, $\Delta P$, or RR will ↑ Minute Ventilation, which therefore ↓ CO$_2$ and ↑ pH |
| | • ↓ VT, $\Delta P$, or RR will ↓ Minute Ventilation, which therefore ↑ CO$_2$ and ↓ pH |

# Additonal Methods of Improving Ventilation

## Respiratory Acidosis
- Allow for permissive hypercapnia
  (allow $CO_2$ to rise and pH to fall to a minimal safe level)
- Increase spontaneous tidal volume
  - Pressure support
  - Short-acting beta agonist
  - Increase ET Tube size
- Decrease mechanical deadspace
  - Use low compliance circuit
  - Cut ET tube shorter
  - Consider tracheotomy
- High frequency ventilation
- Patient positioning (improves V/Q)
- Verify adequate I:E ratio (flow waveform)
- ↓ $CO_2$ production: consider fever, surgeries, trauma, sepsis

## Respiratory Alkalosis
- Decrease pressure support
- Decrease SIMV rate
- Sedation (extreme agitation,, fear, pain, ↑ WOB)
- Add mechanical deadspace (not often used clinically)

**If patient is hyperventilating due to hypoxemia
correct the hypoxemia first**

**Tachypnea is often caused by a metabolic acidosis,
so be aware of ABG**

## ▦ Conventional Ventilation: Weaning

- Weaning strategies vary, but should be aggressive for most neonates.
- Signs that suggest weaning/discontinuation should be initiated:
  - Stable respiratory status (4-8 hours), as evidenced by blood gases, improved P/V loops, etc.
    Spontaneous $\dot{V}E$ of ~ 240-360 mL/kg/min
  - Improvement in CXR
  - Stable hemodynamic status (vasopressors, etc.)
- Parameters should be changed frequently and gradually (not slowly with large decreases)
- Careful monitoring should occur during the weaning phase

**Oxygenation:**
- Decrease $FiO_2$ first, then
- Decrease PEEP if > physiologic (don't drop below 4-5 cm $H_2O$)

**Ventilation**
- If in SIMV, consider ↓ $f$ (see SIMV for notes)
- If Pressure Mode: Decrease PIP until estimated VT is 4-5 cc/kg.
- If Volume Targeted Mode: Decrease target tidal volume, but do not wean below 4-5 cc/kg

**Extubation**
- There are no definitive guidelines. The decision is somewhat subjective.
- Stop feeding 4 hours before extubation
- Place infant on NPPV, NIV NAVA, N-CPAP or HFNC as appropriate. SEE NONINVASIVE CPAP
- Stridor: Consider administering Racemic epinephrine
- Drive: For infants < 34 weeks' gestation, administer methylxanthines (caffeine) if not done previously

## Neurally Adjusted Ventilatory Assist    K
(NAVA, NIV-NAVA)

| Summary | This <u>noninvasive or invasive</u> mode incorporates neural triggering (through a sensor on a specialized nasogastric (NG) catheter - positioned in the esophagus near the diaphragm) with spontaneous breaths that are pressure supported proportionally to the strength of the electrical signal from the diaphragm. |

Neonatal

Ventilation

| Breath Type | | Classified By: | | |
|---|---|---|---|---|
| | | Trigger | Limit | Cycle |
| NAVA | Spontaneous | PT *(Neurally, Press or $\dot{V}$)* | PL *(Neurally)* | PC *(Neurally)* |
| NAVA (PS) | Spontaneous | PT *(Press or $\dot{V}$)* | PL *(Press)* | PC *($\dot{V}$, P, Time)* |
| NAVA BACKUP | Mandatory | MT *(Time)* | ML *(Press)* | MC *(Time)* |
| | Assisted | Assisted breaths will return pt to NAVA | | |

**How It Works**:

Neonatal

- A specialized Nasogastric (NG) tube with an array of electrodes (Edi catheter) is positioned in the esophagus to optimally detect the electrical activity of the diaphragm
- An Edi positioning screen utilizes a 4-channel retrocardiac EKG pattern to assist the clinician on the **proper placement** of the Edi catheter. Correct NG catheter position is demonstrated by the largest p-waves and by the QRS complexes being present in the upper leads and subsequently progressing to minimal or absent p-waves. QRS complexes remain present in the lower leads.
- The Edi signal is superimposed on the retrocardiac EKG as a blue color and should be on the second and third lead but may periodically fluctuate to the upper and lower leads without loss of signal integrity. A trigger level is set. Once the threshold is reached (Edi min + Trigger level), **a breath is initiated**.

Ventilation

- **The ventilator assists the spontaneous breath** of the patient by delivering pressure directly and linearly proprotional to the Edi or neural respiratory drive. Inspiration (pressure delivery) is proportionally maintained until the electrical activity decreases by 30% and the breath is then terminated. This allows the patient to determine inspiratory pressure (or volume), inspiratory and expiratory time, and respiratory rate for each breath.
- The clinician sets a **backup pressure support level** with trigger and cycle off criteria so the patient can flow-trigger the ventilator should the Edi catheter become displaced. Neural respiratory rate and timing can differ from the pneumatic rate and time. This may be caused by well known pneumatic/flow trigger challenges including delayed, false, or missed triggering.
- **In case of apnea** (absent Edi signal and pneumatic triggers that last longer than an adjustable apnea time limit), the ventilator will switch to standard pressure control ventilation (NAVA backup). This adjustable apnea time acts as a minimum rate and can be adjusted from as little as 2 seconds (min. rate 30 breaths/min) to 30 seconds (min. rate 2 breaths /min). **Once the patient starts breathing spontaneously, the ventilator will switch back to a NAVA mode.**

**Indications**:

- Mode is used in neonatal-to-adult populations
- Edi monitoring alone may be done on any patient in any mode of ventilation. This can be used as another respiratory vital sign and gives information about neural respiratory drive, work of breathing, response to sedation, and synchrony in non-NAVA modes.
- Spontaneously breathing patients can be ventilated on NAVA even when having prolonged periods of apnea. Patients should not be paralyzed, overly sedated, or over-ventilated.
- Patients who are dys-synchronous on conventional modes of ventilation

**Proposed Advantages**:

- Reduces work of breathing—less missed patient trigger efforts. Intrinsic PEEP will not affect triggering in NAVA
- Improves synchrony—the patient's neural trigger controls onset, breath size (pressure and volume) and cycling off of each breath. Ventilator synchrony with the patient is an important part of unloading the work of the diaphragm during both inspiration and expiration.
- May reduce need for sedation/paralysis—by allowing the patient to control their own breathing pattern, less sedation may be required
- May improve ventilation—compared to standard methods, by allowing neural triggering, cycling and neurally-adjusted ventilator assistance (e.g., patients with severe airflow impairment)
- May reduce overall peak inspiratory pressures being delivered (patients get the pressure they need for that breath)

**Disadvantages and Risks**:

- Correct placement of the NG catheter is important but easily maintained and monitored. Any significant displacement will interfere with the mode (a backup system as outlined above is in place) and an alarm alerts the provider to reassess catheter position.
- Cannot be used if the respiratory center, phrenic nerve and neuromuscular junction are not intact or are chemically depressed
- The respiratory drive (Edi signal) may not be present if patient is over-ventilated. This may be a result of too high NAVA level or too much backup support.

### Edi Catheter (same catheter for both invasive and noninvasive)

- Edi signal is in microvolts (μv)
- The phrenic nerve activates the diaphragm electrically.  Edi is a representation of this signal.
- There is generally more variability in phases and baseline in infant Edi signals as compared to adult Edi signals
- Increased Edi amplitude (phasic Edi) indicates greater inspiratory effort
- Approved by U.S. FDA as a functioning NG/OG tube

| Edi amplitude increases | Edi amplitude decreases |
|---|---|
| worsening resp. status<br>↓ ventilator assist<br>↓ sedation<br>↑ deadspace<br>↑ ventilatory demand<br>  (e.g., crying, moving, etc.) | improving resp. status<br>↑ ventilator assist<br>↑ sedation<br>↓ deadspace |

| Breath Start (Trigger) | During Breath | Breath End (Cycle) |
|---|---|---|
| Edi Trigger Level (which is set) is reached which initiates | an assist <u>in propor-</u><u>tion to</u> the Edi signal.  This is provided until | the Edi signal has fallen to 70% of its peak value, at which time passive exhalation is allowed |
| Edi Trigger Level | **Pressure delivered (PIP) =**<br><br>NAVA level<br>**x**<br>(Edi signal - Edi min)<br>**+**<br>PEEP | |

**Insertion and Positioning of the Edi Catheter**

| Height | Weight | Edi Catheter Size | Inter-Electrode Distance (IED) |
|--------|--------|-------------------|-------------------------------|
| 45-85 cm | -- | 8 FR 100 cm | 8mm |
| < 55 cm | 1.0 - 2.0 kg | 6 FR 50 cm | 6 mm |
| < 55 cm | 0.5 - 1.5 kg | 6 FR 49 cm | 6 mm |

Neonatal

Ventilation

1. Take NEX Measurement. This is the distance from the bridge of the nose to the earlobe to the xiphoid process.

2. Calculate insertion distance (NEX is measurement from #1)

|  | Nasal (in Y cm) | Oral (in Y cm) |
|--|-----------------|----------------|
| **8 FR 100 cm** | NEX cm x 0.9 + 8 | NEX cm x 0.8 + 8 |
| **6 FR 50 cm** | NEX cm x 0.9 + 3.5 | NEX cm x 0.8 + 3.5 |
| **6 FR 49 cm** | NEX cm x 0.9 + 2.5 | NEX cm x 0.8 + 2.5 |

3. Dip Edi catheter into water - DO NOT USE LUBRICANT
   Insert the catheter to the Y distance from #2

4. Connect catheter to cable

5. Verify positioning of the catheter
   ECG: P, QRS present in top leads
         P waves decrease and disappear; QRS decreases
         If 2nd and 3rd leads are highlighted in blue: secure
         If top leads are highlighted in blue: withdraw to the
            inter-electrode distance (IED)
         If bottom leads are constantly highlighted in blue:
            insert further

**Typical Invasive NAVA Initial Settings** (specific to this mode)

| NAVA level | 0-4 cmH₂O/μV |
|---|---|
| | 1. Start at a NAVA level of 2 cmH₂O/ μV and evaluate the WOB |
| | 2. If ↑ WOB (and associated high Edi peaks) increase the Nava level in 0.5 cmH2O/ μV increments until the patient is comfortable and the Edi peaks are 5-15 μV. Maintain. |
| | 3. If the patient is comfortable and the Edi peaks are < 5 μV, decrease the NAVA level in 0.5 cmH₂O/ μV increments until the Edi peak mostly are > 5 μV or the patient begins to work harder. |
| Trigger Edi | Default = 0.5 μV (range = 0-2 μV) |
| NAVA PS | Ensure adequate PS: Set the PS at the same level as PC in the backup settings |
| Back-Up | ***Ensure Adequate Back-Up:*** <br>**Mode**: Pressure Control <br>**Inspiratory Pressure**: set high enough to move the chest (typically 15-25 cmH₂O) <br>**Rate**: set at 40-60 breaths/min <br>**Inspiratory Time**: 0.3-0.4 second |
| Peak Pressure Limit | Set high enough to allow recruiting breaths (35-40 cmH₂O); ↑ if upper limit is alarming |
| Apnea Time | Set short enough that the patient gets a rescue (backup) breath before any clinical decompensation is noted. This represents minimum ventilator rate. |

**Weaning**

- Once WOB is minimal, Edi peaks < 15 μV, and blood gas is acceptable (pH > 7.25, $PCO_2$ < 60, $O_2$% < 30), decrease NAVA level in 0.5 cmH₂O/ μV increments until the Edi peaks rise, or the patient WOB increases. Attempt 2-3 times/day or as tolerated.
- When at NAVA level of 1 cmH₂O/ μV, consider extubation to NIV NAVA, increasing the NAVA level back to 2 cmH₂O/ μV and titrating to the appropriate level as described above.
- Patients with chronic lung disease may require less frequent and smaller incremental changes in NAVA level.

# Invasive NAVA: How Modes are Automatically Selected[1]

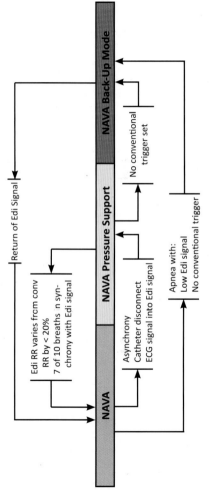

[1]Adapted from Maquet, Inc.: NAVA and NIV NAVA Neonatal Pocket Guide

Neonatal

Ventilation

**Noninvasive NAVA Initial Settings** (specific to this mode)

| NAVA level | 0-4 cmH$_2$O/ µV. Default = 2<br>Start with NAVA level at 2 and adjust as described for invasive NAVA |
|---|---|
| Trigger Edi | Default = 0.5 µV (range = 0-2 µV) |
| Back-Up | **Ensure Adequate Back-Up:**<br>**Mode**: Pressure Control<br>**Inspiratory Pressure**: set high enough to move the chest (typically 20-25 cmH$_2$O)<br>**Rate**: set at 40-60 breaths/min<br>**Inspiratory Time**: 0.35-0.4 second |
| Peak Pressure Limit | Set high enough to allow recruiting breaths (35-40 cmH$_2$O); ↑ if upper limit is alarming |
| Apnea Time | Set short enough that the patient gets a rescue (backup) breath before any clinical decompensation is noted. |

**Weaning**

- Use same approach as with Invasive NAVA
- When NAVA level is 1 cmH$_2$O/uV, consider transition to CPAP

## NAVA Troubleshooting

| Issue | Possible Problem(s) | Possible Correction(s) |
|-------|---------------------|------------------------|
| No or low Edi signal | Over-ventilation<br>Over-sedation<br>Central apnea | Verify muscle relaxants worn off<br>Verify patient's sedation level<br>Verify patient is not hyperventilated<br>Review blood gas/$ErCO_2$ |
| Stays in NAVA (Backup) mode<br>(no neural or pneumatic trigger) | Over-ventilation<br>Over-sedation<br>Central apnea | Decrease ventilation and monitor<br>Decrease sedation and monitor<br>Consider changing ventilator mode |
| Stays in NAVA (PS) mode<br>Alarm: Pneumatic-Edi out of synch | Most commonly from a large air leak | Make the flow trigger less sensitive<br>Reintubate with a larger ET tube<br>Change to NIV NAVA used invasively |
| | **Specific cases of asynchrony:**<br>• Edi RR differs from pneumatic RR with > 25% for at least 5 seconds (calculated RR based on last 20 seconds)<br>• Edi TI/TTOT > 0.5 seconds (calculated over last 20 seconds)<br>• Edi catheter disconnected<br>• EKG leakage through Edi signal | Check Edi signal<br>Ensure proper catheter position<br>Troubleshoot in this order:<br>1. ↓ pneumatic trigger setting<br>2. Adjust (↑ or ↓) the Edi trigger in increments of 0.1 uV<br>3. Adjust inspiratory cycle off setting |

| | | |
|---|---|---|
| Respiratory acidosis in infants with apnea of prematurity who are experiencing multiple apneic episodes per minute | • Insufficient backup support when patient is in the NAVA (backup) mode <br> • Apnea time is too long | Increase set backup rate and/or PC above PEEP <br><br> Shorten apnea time |
| *Edi Monitoring not active* message | NAVA mode is activated without the Edi module being connected | Connect and perform the Edi Module test |
| *Edi Module disconnected* message <br> *Edi Module error* message | Edi module is not properly installed | Reinsert module and perform the Edi Module test |
| *Check Edi catheter position* message | Edi catheter not in appropriate position | Check Edi catheter positioning screen and reposition Edi catheter as needed |
| *Peak Inspiratory Pressure* alarm | Peak pressure limit set too low | Assess patient <br> Increase peak pressure limit |
| Edi min is consistently higher than 3.0 | This may be an indication that additional PEEP is needed | Consider increasing PEEP |

# ◼ High Frequency Ventilation Strategies
### See following pages for HFOV and HFJV details

| Factors | HFOV | HFFI[1] | HFJV |
|---------|------|---------|------|
| Operation | Piston moves back and forth | Interruption of flow source | Delivers pulsed jets (proximal end of ET Tube) |
| Limit | Pressure | Pressure | Pressure |
| Tidal Volume | < deadspace | > deadspace | < deadspace |
| Hertz Rates/min | 3-15 Hz 180-900 | 2-28 Hz 120-1680 | 4-11 Hz 240-660 |
| Exhalation | Active | Passive or Assisted | Passive |
| Gas Flow | Sinusoidal | Helical | Helical |
| Conventional ventilator required? | Works independently | Usually Requires | Usually Requires |

[1] High Frequency Flow Interruptors are used primarily during studies in labs but are included here for comparison sake.

**Clinical Notes:**

**High-frequency Conventional Ventilation:** The use of rates up to 2.5 Hz (150 breaths/min) was explored, but are not used clinically today.

**There are two primary goals:**
1. Open the lungs (open lung ventilation)
2. Provide small, non-damaging tidal volumes

## Indications
**Prophylactic (protective):**

Thresholds and Guidelines vary. For example:
- VLBW from delivery
- Known pulmonary hypoplasia
- Severe abdominal distension requiring ventilation

**Early Intervention (usually RDS):**
- Increasing $FIO_2$ despite optimal mean airway pressure
- $V_T$ > 6 cc/kg
- Deterioration of ABGs without improvement following ventilator changes, despite optimal mPAW and $V_T$
- Air leak syndromes
- Persistent pulmonary hypertension of the newborn

## Contraindications
- Obstructive lung disease processes - use caution

## High Frequency Oscillatory Ventilation (HFOV)

| Summary | Often referred to as "the oscillator." |
|---|---|
| | A Mean Airway Pressure (mPAW) is set to keep the airways/alveoli open (like CPAP does), and then very small breaths (which are less than deadspace) are delivered at very high rates |
| | Inspiration and exhalation are both active (this is unusual as exhalation is passive in most modes of ventilation) |

**Neonatal**

**Ventilation**

**Ventilators**:

Sensormedics 3100A: stand-alone oscillator with diaphragm used in neonates/infants

Sensormedics 3100B: stand-alone oscillator with diaphragm approved for > 35 kg

| Breath Type | Classified By: | | |
|---|---|---|---|
| | Trigger | Limit | Cycle |
| Mandatory *(Controlled)* | MT *(Time)* | PL *(Pressure)* | MC *(Time)* |

*Note that while this technically classifies a breath, HFOV does not utilize conventional breaths for the majority of the alveoli. These small breaths theoretically use passive gas diffusion, pendelluft, assymetric velocity profiles, turbulence, and other mechanisms of gas flow at very high rates to distribute and exchange gases.

**Definitions**

| | |
|---|---|
| **mPAW** | Mean Airway Pressure, which directly affects Oxygenation. The maximum possible is 55-60 cmH$_2$O |
| **Bias Flow** | Flow of gases through circuit which maintains set mean airway pressure. Increasing bias flow will enable an increase in mPAW |
| **Power** | Controls electrical current level applied to motor. This <u>setting</u> on the oscillator alters the $\Delta$P which effects CO$_2$ elimination |
| **Amplitude (delta-P)** | **Primary determinant of CO$_2$ elimination** HFOV ventilation = $f$ x V$_T^2$ Conventional ventilation = $f$ x V$_T$ Changes in V$_t$ affect CO$_2$ more drastically than changes in $f$ |
| **Hertz Hz (Frequency)** | **Secondary determinant of CO$_2$ elimination** Number of times the piston moves fully forward and fully backward (1 inhalation + 1 exhalation) Hertz x 60 = Cycles/minute Hertz is inversely proportional to volume (the higher the Hz, the lower the oscillating volumes) |
| **Inspiratory Time** | The amount of time the piston is in the forward motion This is set as a % on oscillator (usually 33%) |
| **Expiratory Time** | Backward movement of the piston Unlike most modes of ventilation, exhalation is active |
| **Chest Wiggle Factor (CWF)** | An informal manner of assessing volume displacement (amplitude/power) |

## HFOV (Oscillator)
## Suggested Initial Settings (based on 3100A)
(non-disease specific)

| | | |
|---|---|---|
| **Primary Oxygenation** | **MAP** | Direct: 8-10 cmH₂O<br>From Conventional:<br>    2-4 cmH₂O above<br>    conventional MAP |
| | **Inspiratory Time** | 33% |
| | **FIO₂** | Match from conventional |
| **（middle section）** | **Power**<br>**1-10** | < 2.0 kg    Power 2.5<br>2.0-2.5 kg    Power 3.0<br>2.5-4.0 kg    Power 4.0<br>4.0-5.0 kg    Power 5.0<br>5.0-10.0 kg    Power 6.0<br>> 20 kg    Power 7.0 |
| | **Delta-P (ΔP)**<br>**Amplitude**<br>*ΔP is set indirectly*<br>*by changing power* | Set for presence of chest<br>wiggle in the neonate (use<br>values in Power - above - for<br>initial setting) |
| | **Hertz (Hz)** | Preterm    10-15 Hz<br>Term        8-10 Hz<br><br>Both depend on lung disease.<br>Use higher for restrictive dis-<br>orders; lower for obstructive<br>disorders. |
| **Other** | **Bias Flow**<br>**(L/min)** | 8-15 L/min pre-term<br>10-20 L/min term or<br>            near-term<br><br>Too low: can't reach MAP<br>Too high: prevents full<br>        exhalation (↑ CO₂) |

## Special Note on Ventilation with HFOV:

Power and $\Delta$P are interconnected. Power is a setting on the oscillator which controls $\Delta$P. $\Delta$P is a measurement, and is thus set primarily by the Power setting.

Some clinicians target a specific power setting, allowing $\Delta$P to change in response to compliance/resistance changes in the patient. Other clinicians target a specific $\Delta$P and thus will regularly alter the power setting to ensure the target $\Delta$P.

↑ Power results in ↑ $\Delta$P (↑ ventilation)
↓ Power results in ↓ $\Delta$P (↓ ventilation)

# HFOV: Managing and Monitoring

## Primary Methods for Adjusting Oxygenation

| #1 Optimize Mean Airway Pressure |
| --- |
| Oxygenation on the oscillator is primarily targeted by using mPAW.<br>CXR: Goal is convex diaphragms, minimal atelectasis, normal-sized heart. 8-9 ribs posteriorly above diaphragm is used (but may be misleading) |

| #2 Titrate FIO₂ |
| --- |
| The goal is to maintain a safe O₂% whenever possible. Optimizing mPAW has greater benefit in the long-term. |

## Primary Methods for Adjusting Ventilation

| Problem: ↑ PaCO₂ = underventilated | |
| --- | --- |
| #1 Power/ΔP | Increase ΔP to increase the amplitude (~ size of the breath) |
| #2 Frequency[1] | ↓ Hertz<br>This is counter-intuitive!<br>Reducing frequency ↑ ventilation |
| #3 Inspiratory Time | Leave at 33%<br>Some clinicians recommend increasing Inspiratory Time to 50% (no higher) for ~10% increase in V$_T$ |

| Problem: ↓ PaCO₂ = overventilated | |
| --- | --- |
| #1 Power/ΔP | Decrease ΔP but ensure adequate chest wiggle |
| #2 Frequency[1] | ↑ Hertz<br>This is counter-intuitive!<br>Increasing Frequency ↓ ventilation |

[1] Hertz is rarely changed when it is acceptable for patient size and lung disease.

### Clinical Notes

- An initial CXR should be obtained within 1-2 hours to determine over- and underexpansion based upon heart size, diaphragms, and atelectasis.
- Suctioning (discouraged for first 24-hours unless clinically indicated):
  - diminished chest wall wiggle
  - increasing $CO_2$
  - decreasing $PO_2$
  - visible or audible secretions
- Some clinicians stop the piston (start/stop button) during suctioning. If pressure is "dumped" during suctioning, it may be necessary to re-pressurize the circuit (Reset button), and then start piston (Start/Stop button).

### Weaning HFOV

Wean $FiO_2$ as tolerated to target $SpO_2/PO_2$

- Wean mPAW and $\Delta P$ - monitor $SpO_2/PO_2$ and CXR closely
  - Wean mPAW in 1-2 cm $H_2O$ increments
  - Wean $\Delta P$ in 2-4 cm $H_2O$ increments
- Consider extubating to NPPV or N-CPAP when:
  - mPAW = 7-9 cm $H_2O$
  - CXR is clear (or nearly clear)
  - $FIO_2$ < 30-40% (0.30 - 0.40)
  - Infant is noted to be breathing comfortably
  - Amplitude will usually be < 20

Note: Transition to conventional mechanical ventilation is not necessary, thought is common practice in neonatal and pediatric populations

## HFOV Troubleshooting

*(see manufacturer documentation for a more complete list)*

### Technical Troubleshooting

| | |
|---|---|
| **Oscillator stopped with no other alarms** | • Ensure circuit has been re-pressurized (reset button) before starting piston<br>• Ensure ΔP is > 6 cmH₂O<br>• Ensure oscillator piston is centered |
| **Unable to maintain Mean Airway Pressure** | Check for leaks -<br>• check all mushroom valves (cap diaphragm)<br>• check water trap stopcock (ensure screwed in)<br>• Check humidifier - with some therapeutic modalities, 1-way valves may be needed (e.g. iNO)<br>• Check ET Tube<br><br>Check bias flow rate - may be insufficient |
| **Mean Airway Pressure not maintaining at desired value** | • Pt may be spontaneously breathing (less likely with pre-term infants) |
| **Will not Meet Circuit Calibration** | • Check for leaks<br>• Ensure adequate flowmeter setting |
| **Low Pressure alarm** | • Consider any break in circuit<br>• Check mushroom valves, replace if necessary |

## Clinical Troubleshooting and Considerations

<table>
<tr><td rowspan="1">Neonatal</td><td>Increasing Respiratory Acidosis</td><td><ul><li>Decreased ET Tube diameter</li><li>Mucous plug</li><li>Pulmonary edema</li><li>Decreased Power or Amplitude settings</li><li>Decrease IT &lt; 33%</li><li>Decreased Compliance</li><li>Increased Hertz</li></ul></td></tr>
<tr><td rowspan="5">Ventilation</td><td>Patient Transport</td><td><ul><li>Avoid transport if possible - perform procedures and tests at bedside</li></ul>If necessary:<ul><li>Clamp ET Tube with piston stopped, but HFOV on (circuit remains pressurized)</li><li>Bag pt with self-inflating manual resuscitator with PEEP valve (approximate mPAW from HFOV settings and bag with small, rapid breaths)</li><li>Unclamp ET tube and provide high quality ventilations</li><li>Strongly consider setting up an oscillator at destination—or a high PEEP strategy to maintain recruitment of lungs</li></ul></td></tr>
<tr><td>Chest Wiggle Decreased</td><td><ul><li>ET tube moved or obstructed</li><li>Pneumothorax (unilateral ↓)</li><li>ET tube right mainstem (↓ wiggle on left side)</li></ul></td></tr>
<tr><td>Increased mPaw, amplitude</td><td><ul><li>ET Tube obstruction (mucous)</li><li>Secretions</li><li>Bronchospasm</li><li>Rule out tension PTX</li></ul></td></tr>
<tr><td>Hypotension<br>↑ CVP</td><td><ul><li>Consider pulmonary overdistension</li></ul></td></tr>
</table>

## High Frequency Jet Ventilation
(HFJV)

| Summary | Often referred to as "the jet." Works as a flow interrupter (uses a pinch tube and valve), delivering a high pressure pulse of gas via a special ET Tube adapter. Used in tandem with a conventional ventilator (which delivers PEEP, FIO₂, sigh breaths) |
|---|---|

**M**

**Ventilators:**
Bunnell Life Pulse

|  | Classified By: | | |
|---|---|---|---|
| **Breath Type** | **Trigger** | **Limit** | **Cycle** |
| **Mandatory** *(Controlled)* | MT *(Time)* | PL *(Pressure)* | MC *(Time)* |

### Controls

PIP
Rate
Jet Valve Time On (Inspiratory Time)

### Monitored

| **PIP** | averaged maximum airway pressures |
|---|---|
| **PEEP** | averaged minimum airway pressures |
| **MAP** | averaged pressures from total pressure waveform includes spontaneous breaths and conventional ventilator |
| **ΔP** | difference between PIP and PEEP (reflects tidal volume) |
| **Servo Pressure** | Unitless number - driving pressure that controls the flow required to meet PIP, Rate, and TI on Jet |

## HFJV (Jet)
## Suggested Initial Settings (based on Bunnell)
(non-disease specific)

**When converting to HFJV, take care to maintain stable mPAW as much as possible**

| | | |
|---|---|---|
| **Set directly on Jet Ventilator** | Peak Inspiratory Pressure (PIP) | *Ventilating well:*<br>  From vent: PIP - 2 cm H$_2$O<br>  From HFOV: PIP - 2 cm H$_2$O<br>*Not ventilating well:*<br>  Match PIP from vent/HFOV |
| | Rate (Hz) | 420 breaths/min (7 Hz)<br>Decrease if risk of air-trapping<br>*Rate is changed in increments of 1 Hz (60 breaths)* |
| | Jet Valve On Time (I-Time) | 0.02 sec |
| **Set directly on Ventilator (running with jet)** | PEEP | Add 2 cmH$_2$O PEEP when transitioning from just ventilator |
| | Rate | Air leak: 0 breaths/min<br>RDS: 0 breaths/min<br><br>*Use rate if there are areas of atelectasis and also areas of hyperexpansion. Conventional rate should not exceed 6 breaths/min* |
| | PIP | PEEP + ~6 cmH$_2$O |
| | I-Time | 0.4 sec or less |

# HFJV: Managing and Monitoring

## Primary Methods for Improving Oxygenation
*Guiding Principal: Decrease conventional ventilation whenever possible. Ensure adequate PEEP in all circumstances.*

**Problem**: Under-oxygenated

| #1:  Check for over-expansion on CXR | |
|---|---|
| If over-expansion is noted, decrease PEEP. | |
| **#2:  Conventional Ventilator changes** | |
| **Increase PEEP** | Increase in small increments<br>Ensure no over-distention |
| **Increase $f$** | Do not exceed 6 breaths/min |
| **Increase PIP/VT** | Cautiously consider with goal of preventing lung injury<br>Use conventional ventilation PIP that approximates a normal tidal volume |
| **Increase TI** | Increases mPAW |
| **#3.  Jet Ventilator changes** | |
| **Increase Rate** | Increase by ~1 Hz<br>Rate > 420 is seldom useful for $CO_2$ elimination<br>Be cautious of air-trapping (I:E ratio is shortened) |
| **Increase PIP** | Do not cause hyperventilation |

## Primary Methods for Adjusting Ventilation

**Neonatal**

| Problem:  Increased PaCO₂ (under-ventilated) | |
|---|---|
| **#1 Increase Jet PIP** | PaO₂ acceptable: ↑ Jet PIP<br>PaO₂ unacceptable: Check PEEP |
| **#2 Lower PEEP** | If air leaks or over-expansion (heart vessels compressed): ↓ PEEP |
| **#3 Increase Jet Rate** | Consider increasing by 40-80 breaths<br>*less effective than changing PIP* |
| **#4 Change conventional ventilator** | Decrease rate, PIP, TI |

**Ventilation**

| Problem: Decreased PaCO₂ (over-ventilated) | |
|---|---|
| **#1 Decrease Jet PIP** | Caution:  consider raising PEEP to avoid critical loss of mPAW |
| **#2 Decrease Jet Rate** | Minimum rate: 240 breaths/min |

## How to use Servo Pressure:

- Servo Pressure is the driving pressure that automatically regulates flow. It can be used to monitor changes in patient status (compliance, resistance), similar to, though inversely, the PIP.
- The specific servo pressure is less important than how it trends. It is best to establish a baseline by comparing a good ABG with the corresponding servo pressure.

| Servo P ↑ from baseline | Servo P ↓ from baseline |
|---|---|
| Disconnected tube<br>Air leak | Secretions (suctioning needed)<br>ET Tube obstructed<br>Right mainstem intubation<br>Tension Pneumothorax |
| Improving compliance<br>Improving resistance | Worsening compliance<br>Worsening resistance |

## Clinical Notes:

- There is some evidence to suggest secretions may be mobilized during Jet ventilation. Be prepared to suction.
- Suctioning can be done by placing the Jet in stand-by, or by suctioning (closed or open system) with the Jet running. If suctioning with Jet running: as long as "Ready" light is on, the PIP will be maintained despite the "Loss of PIP" alarm. If PIP is lost during suctioning, press "Enter."

## Weaning the Jet

- Discontinue the conventional ventilator rate, if set.
- Decrease FiO₂ until below 30%
  Continue to wean Jet PIP until in mid-teens
  Maintain Vent PIP (this will cause interruptions in the Jet)
- Now add conventional ventilator support as Jet PIP is weaned
  Goal: Jet PIP ≤ 15; Vent Rate 15-20
  Then: Trial on Conventional Vent by placing Jet on stand-by
- Extubate to NPPV or N-CPAP when:
  - mPAW 7-9 cm H₂O (Jet PIP will usually be < 20)
  - FiO₂ < 30-40% (0.30 - 0.40)
  - Infant is noted to be breathing comfortably

## HFJV Troubleshooting

*(see manufacturer documentation for a more complete list)*

| | |
|---|---|
| **The majority of alarms occur due to kinked, obstructed, or disconnected tubes.** | Check tubing early in process, then as appropriate unkink tubes, reconnect tubes, and clear obstructions. |
| **Pauses during operation** | This is usually a purge of the pressure monitoring tube - occurs at higher set rates, usually about 1x/15 sec |
| **Jet valve fault** | • Replace the patient box<br>• Change out ventilator |
| **Cannot Meet PIP**<br>*activates when the monitored PIP has not been stable. May also mean servo pressure has maxed out.* | • Is pt breathing spontaneously, crying, coughing, etc.?<br>• Consider suctioning<br>• Check for bronchospasm<br>• If servo P has reached max (20 PSI) before reaching the PIP, pt may be too large to be ventilated with Jet<br>• Increase TI if jet is working properly (normally the shorter the TI, the better. The lowest possible is 0.20)<br>• Check humidity (over-humidification)<br>• Ensure pressure monitoring tube is pointed up<br>• Check for leaks<br>• Check the pinch valve |

# 5 Neonatal Procedures

CONTENTS

Neonatal

Procedures

# ■ Neonatal Airway Management

Neonatal

**Manual Resuscitation**

Three main ways to provide bag/mask or bag/artificial airway ventilation:

| | |
|---|---|
| **T-piece resuscitator** | Has a PIP and a PEEP<br>Occluding the port provides a positive pressure breath<br>Requires a flow of gas |
| **Flow Inflating Bag** | Requires a flow of gas and a good seal to provide ventilation |
| **Self-inflating bag** | Self-inflates with or without gas flow. |

Procedures

- Manual resuscitators in NICU need to be run via an Air/O₂ blender, at the lowest Oxygen percentage to achieve minimum oxygenation goals
- There is insufficient evidence to support any specific type of resuscitator
- A flow-inflating bag should NOT be the only resuscitator brought on a transport (if a pressurized gas source becomes unavailable, such as if a cylinder is empty, there will be no way to ventilate the infant)
- Pressure-relief valves and pressure manometers should be integrated into the set-up, either as part of equipment design, or appropriately connected in-line
- Visible chest rise is the best confirmation of adequate ventilation

# ■ Bag Mask Ventilation Positioning in Neonates

Correct:

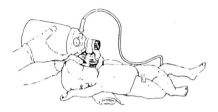

Overextension:

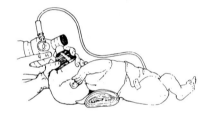

Overflexion:

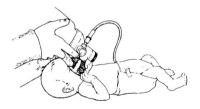

Reprinted with permission from Schreiner, R. and Kisling, J. *Practical Neonatal Respiratory Care.* Copyright 1982 by Raven Press.

## ▦ Suctioning

### Indications

*Suctioning should be done when indicated, not on a set schedule*

- Evidence of secretions: visible secretions in tube, audible coarse breath sounds, or ↓ breath sounds
- Deterioration of vital signs: changes in respiratory pattern, ↑ WOB, tachypnea, apnea, tachycardia or bradycardia
- Changes in oxygenation or ventilation: labile $SpO_2$, skin color changes (pale, cyanotic, dusky), Respiratory Acidosis on ABG, ↑ PIP on ventilator

| Choose appropriate catheter size | Weight (grams) | Size (French) |
|---|---|---|
| | < 1000 | 5 |
| | < 2000 | 6 |
| | < 3000 | 6-8 |
| | > 3000 | 6-8 |

| Pre-oxygenation / Pre-ventilation | • Routine pre-oxygenation is discouraged in neonates. If critical oxygenation, consider increasing $O_2$ by 10-20% from baseline<br>• Avoid hyperventilation which increases risk of air leaks |
|---|---|
| Set vacuum pressure | -60 to -80 mm Hg |
| Suction | • Note length of ET tube, including adapter. The catheter should not be advanced more than 1 cm beyond this distance.<br>• Using asceptic technique, gently insert catheter to pre-determined length. If cough is noted, it is likely that catheter has been inserted too deep<br>• Apply suction while withdrawing catheter. Limit attempt to 10 seconds. Limit number of attempts. |

## Intubation

**Indications**
- HR < 100 bpm after 30 seconds of ventilating effectively -or-
  No detectable heartbeat
  Apnea despite ventilating effectively
- Inability to effectively ventilate
- Certain congenital anomalies

| Choose appropriate supplies | • Uncuffed ET Tubes (various sizes recommended, see chart below)<br>• Miller (straight) Laryngoscope blades (various sizes recommended, see chart below)<br>• End-tidal $CO_2$ detector (colorimetric or volumetric)<br>• Suction<br>• ET Tube stabilization equipment (tape, etc.)<br>• Resuscitator bag (and t-piece resuscitator, if available) with various masks<br>• Laryngeal Mask Airway (LMA) |
|---|---|

**Airway Insertion Selection[1]**

| Weight[2] (grams) | Gestation (weeks) | Laryngo-scope Blade | ET Tube Size (mm ID) | Depth at Lip (cm) |
|---|---|---|---|---|
| 500-600 | 23-24 | 00 | 2.5 | 5.5 |
| 700-800 | 25-26 | 00 | 2.5 | 6.0 |
| 900-1000 | 27-29 | 00 | 2.5 - 3.0 | 6.5 |
| 1000-1400 | 30-32 | 0 | 3.0 | 7.0 |
| 1500-1800 | 33-34 | 0 | 3.0 | 7.5 |
| 1900-2400 | 35-37 | 0 | 3.0 - 3.5 | 8.0 |
| 2500-3100 | 38-40 | 0-1 | 3.5 | 8.5 |
| 3200-4200 | 41-43 | 0-1 | 3.5 - 4.0 | 9.0 |

[1] Information presented is based on Kempley, ST, Moreiras, JW, Petrone, FL. *Resuscitation* 2008:77(3). It is consistent with current national guidelines, including STABLE and NRP.

[2] When weight is known, use that first. When weight is unknown, use estimated gestation

| Procedure | • Correct position for intubating is at the head of patient<br>• Infant should in a neutral, supine position. Do NOT hyperextend airway<br>• Manually ventilate as needed, but use caution with pressures and supplemental oxygen<br>• Hold scope in LEFT hand, open mouth with fingers of RIGHT hand<br>• Insert blade over tongue, pushing it towards the LEFT. Slowly advance the blade until the vocal cords come into view. Maintain upward, not rotated, position with the laryngoscope.<br>• If vocal cords are not visible, consider gentle cricoid pressure<br>• Using the RIGHT hand, insert the ET Tube on the RIGHT side and advance down until mark on ET tube advances through vocal cords. See depth information below.<br>• Immediately check placement using depth marking, ETCO$_2$, monitoring chest rise, and auscultating. Confirm placement with X-ray. |
|---|---|
| Tube Insertion Depth | • **Nasal-to-Tragus Length (NTL)**<br>  • Measure the centimeters between nasal septum and ear tragus (the ear flap above the ear lobe)<br>  • Insertion Depth = NTL cm + 1 cm<br>• **Tochen's Rule (7-8-9)\***<br>  • depth (cm) = 6 + (weight in kilograms)<br>  • **\*May overestimate depth, particularly in neonates < 750g, but may still be considered per NRP**<br>• Verify tube position by Chest X-Ray, with the goal of ET Tube tip being between T1-T2 |

# ▨ Transillumination

**Indications:** Suspicion of pneumothorax or pneumomediastinum

**Procedure:**
- A high-intensity light (such as a pen light) is placed against the chest wall in a darkened room.
- If air is present, the chest wall will light up (illuminate)
- If not an emergency, confirm findings with a CXR. If emergent, intervene without waiting for radiographic confirmation.

## student tip

Maintaining a mastery of anatomy and physiology is one key to excelling as a clinician. Keep these points in mind for infants:
- Larynx is more anterior and cephalad
- Tongue is relatively large
- Cricoid ring is the narrowest portion of airway (more funnel-shaped)
- Epiglottis is longer, stiffer, protrudes at about 45 degrees

# Blood Gas Sampling

## ■ Blood Gas Sampling

*Good for small sample draws (< 1 mL)*

**Puncture Sites**
- Heel (posterio-lateral, or medial). This is preferred site in preterm infants.
- Fingers and toes (lateral aspects of distal phalanges) - both older infants and children

**Procedure**

| Arterialize Site | • Choose site that is lateral or medial of the heel<br>• Warm puncture site (optional) to no more than 40° C for 5-10 min using an approved device to avoid burns |
|---|---|
| Infection Control | • Perform hand hygiene<br>• Don gloves<br>• Wipe chosen site with antiseptic, and allow to dry<br>• Use sterile gauzes |
| Puncture | • Puncture with a lancing incision device.<br>• Discard first drop of blood (wipe with gauze)<br>• Collect sample into collection device (such as a capillary tube)<br>• It may be necessary to squeeze gently to allow for blood flow; excessive squeezing may result in hemolysis<br>• Elevate puncture site, applying pressure with gauze pad until bleeding stops |

## Capillary Blood Gas Sampling for Neonatal/Pediatric Patients
## AARC Expert Panel Reference-Based Guidelines

| Description | Hazards / Complications |
|---|---|

**Description**

Capillary blood sample to estimate pH and $PaCO_2$ (It is of little value in estimating $PaO_2$)

**Indications**

Abnormal noninvasive monitor readings ($PtcO_2$, $PetCO_2$, $SpO_2$)

Arterial ABG access is not available

Assessment of therapeutic modalities

Monitoring of a disease process

Patient status change (based on history or physical assessment)

**Contraindications**

Absolute:

Patients less than 24 hrs. old

Site locations not to be used -

Areas of infection

Cyanotic or poorly perfused

Fingers of neonates

Heel (posterior curvature or callused)

Inflamed, swollen or edematous tissue

Peripheral arteries

Previous puncture sites

When direct analysis of arterial blood is needed

Relative:

Hypotension

Peripheral vasoconstriction

Polycythemia

**Hazards / Complications**

Artery laceration

Bleeding

Bone calcification

Bruising

Burns

Inappropriate patient management from reliance of $PcO_2$

Infection (patient or caregiver)

Nerve damage

Pain

Scarring

**Limitations of method**

Inadequate warming of site

Second puncture may be needed

Undue squeezing of puncture site

Variability of $PcO_2$

**Limitations of validity**

Air contamination

Analysis of sample delayed (> 15 min., room temp; > 60 min., iced)

Clotting

Sample quantity insufficient

**Monitoring**

Monitor and document:

Date, time and sampling site

Ease (or difficulty) of obtaining sample

CONTINUED NEXT PAGE

| (Capillary Sampling continued from previous page) | |
|---|---|
| Free flow of blood (without 'milking') | **Frequency** |
| Oxygen administration (device, FiO$_2$ or flow) | No prescribed frequency |
| | Dependent upon indications and clinical status of the patient |
| **Patient -** | |
| Adverse reactions or complications | **Infection Control** |
| Clinical appearance | Aseptic technique |
| Level of activity or position | Universal precautions |
| Puncture site appearance | |
| Respiratory rate | |
| Temperature | |
| Results of analysis | |
| Sample contamination (air or clot) | |
| Values of noninvasive monitors (PtcO$_2$, PetCO$_2$, SpO$_2$) | |
| Ventilator settings | |

Adapted from AARC Clinical Practice Guideline, Respiratory Care, Vol. 46 (5), 2001.

# ▤ Arterial Blood Gas Sampling

*Good for larger sample draws, when an arterial blood sample is critical, or when other lines/methods are unavailable*

## Puncture Sites
- Radial artery

## Contraindications
- Coagulation defect
- Inadequate collateral circulation
- Infection in sample area
- Circulatory compromise

## Procedure

| Locate puncture site | • Extend wrist (do not hyperextend)<br>• Palpate artery (or transilluminate) |
|---|---|
| Perform Modified Allen's Test | • Elevate hand, apply pressure to radial and ulnar arteries, massage palm, then release ulnar artery.<br>• Color returns in:<br>  < 10 sec = adequate circulation<br>  > 10 sec = inadequate circulation |
| Puncture | • Use antiseptic on puncture site<br>• Puncture <u>against the flow of blood</u> using a 15- to 45-degree angle<br>  *more shallow - smaller infants<br>• Advance needle slowly<br>• If resistance is met (bone) or no blood flashes, withdraw slowly (but don't remove), then re-palpate and slowly advance again<br>• Once there is blood flow attach syringe to tubing and aspirate very gently<br>• Remove needle and apply firm pressure at the puncture site until bleeding stops |

# ◼ Umbilical Artery Catheter (UAC)

### Indications

Respiratory failure or cardiovascular collapse in the newborn infant where percutaneous attempts for vascular access have failed.

### Purpose

- Frequent ABG sampling or $SaO_2$ monitoring
- Continuous BP monitoring
- Infusions of parenteral fluids and medications

> **Note**: Umbilical catheters should be removed as soon as clinically appropriate.

### Equipment

- Antiseptic (povidine-iodine) solution
- Sterile drapes, gauze pads, mask, gown and gloves
- Hemostats, scissors, scalpel, needles, sutures (3.0 silk)
- 10 mL syringe filled with normal saline, 3-way stopcock.
- Heparinized infusion solution (1 unit/ml)
- Umbilical catheter (3.5 FR < 1500 gm, 5.0 Fr > 1500 gm)

# Umbilical Artery Catheter Placement Procedure

1. Place patient supine and restrain limbs if necessary
2. Ensure proper oxygenation, ventilation and thermoregulation
3. Monitor vital signs during procedure
4. Use sterile procedure to include hand washing, gloves, gown, mask
5. Prepare catheter. Attach to stopcock and syringe
6. Prepare cord stump and surrounding area with antiseptic and drape
7. Place 3.0 silk tie around base of cord to make a purse string. Do not tighten
8. Cut cord 1-2 cm above abdominal wall
9. Locate vessels:
   2 arteries (thick-walled and round)
   1 vein (thin-walled and oval)
10. Dilate umbilical artery with small curved forceps
11. Insert catheter and advance gently and slowly under constant tension to overcome resistance where the artery bends. A pulsatile blood return should appear after the second bend.
12. Advance catheter desired distance:
    Low position — L3-4
    High position — T8
    Note:   Advance catheter an extra 1-2 cm to allot for the stump height. Remember it is possible to withdraw catheter if advanced too far (after x-ray verification), but it cannot be advanced later if not in far enough (a new catheter would be required).
13. Confirm blood flow at final point
14. Tighten purse string knot
15. Secure catheter
16. Infuse heparin solution (unless contraindicated)
17. Verify position with abdominal x-ray
18. Document

| Complications to Watch For |
|---|

Air embolization

Hemorrhage (vessel perforation, catheter dislodgement or leaks/disconnects)

Hypertension

Infection

Necrotizing enterocolitis

Thrombus formation

Vasospasm — arterial supply to one leg is compromised. Try warming contralateral leg. Remove catheter if blood supply does not improve adequately.

Caution: rapid withdrawal of blood sample may compromise cerebral blood flow (withdraw over a 40 second period)

## Umbilical Venous Catheter (UVC)

### Indications
Immediate access to a vein is needed for an emergency situation (ex. delivery room resuscitation)

### Equipment and Procedure
Same as UAC placement except the umbilical vein is catheterized and the tip is placed in the inferior vena cava/right atrial junction

Avoid placement in right atrium, liver, or portal venous system

# Medical Gases

## Oxygen Administration in the Neonate

### Indications

- Hypoxemia: SpO₂ < 90%
  PaO₂ < 50-60 mm Hg
- Resuscitation (based on AHA/AAP/ILCOR 2015 guidelines)

| Gestational Age | Heart Rate | |
|---|---|---|
| | **HR > 60** | **HR < 60 after 90 sec of resuscitation** |
| < 35 weeks | 21-30 % | Increase to 100% until HR is in normal range |
| ≥ 35 weeks | Room Air | |

- Cyanosis: Central or Generalized
  - Use the minimum concentration that causes cyanosis to resolve, and then regulate per PaO₂/SpO₂
  - Cyanosis may be a late and unreliable sign. It is often not present until PaO₂ 32-42 mm Hg (fetal heme) or 42-53 mm Hg (mature heme). It also varies by ambient light, Hgb/Hct levels, perfusion, skin complexion, etc.

### Hyperoxia

There is a fine balance between the consequences of hypoxia versus hyperoxia, particularly in the premature neonate. Clinicians must treat hyperoxia as seriously as hypoxia in this population.

Potential effects of hyperoxia:
1. Oxygen causes vasoconstriction
   - Retinopahy of Prematurity (ROP) results from repeated or prolonged vasoconstriction to the retina, leading to blindness
   - Premature closure of ductus arteriosus in some heart defects
2. Oxygen releases cytokines, initiating an inflammatory response
   - Bronchopulmonary dysplasia

### Recommendations for O₂ Therapy (AAP/ACOG Summary)[1]

- Supplemental oxygen should be administered for specific indications (cyanosis, $PaO_2$, $SpO_2$)
- Clinical assessment of physical signs can be used in the short-term, but not for ongoing oxygen therapy
- For acute care, pH and $PaCO_2$ should be measured in addition to $PaO_2$
- Oxygen should be ordered to a stated range (maintain $SpO_2$ within specific limits). For preterm infants this is somewhere around 91%-95%.
- Continuous $SpO_2$ combined with periodic measurement of $PaO_2$ is the preferred method of monitoring O₂ therapy. Correlate $SpO_2$ with $PaO_2$ when infant is unstable (as often as every 8-24 hours)
- The combined use of $SpO_2$ (or, more rarely, $tcpO_2$) and capillary arterialized blood gases can guide O₂ therapy with the knowledge that $tcpO_2$ does not accurately estimate $PaO_2$. Do not allow $SpO_2$ to be over 95% in these cases, particulary with preterm infants.

[1] Summarized from: *Guidelines for Perinatal Care*, 7th edition, American Academy of Pediatrics, American College of Obstetric and Gynecologists, 2012

## Neonatal Oxygen Delivery Devices

*Except at the lowest flows, oxygen for neonates (especially premies) should be heated and humidified*

| Device | Liter Flow | Notes |
|--------|-----------|-------|
| **Nasal Cannula (NC)** | 0.1 - 6 L/min (variable) | • Best practice is to run a nasal cannula with a blender<br>• O₂% is variable based upon minute ventilation, blender settings<br>• May create PEEP-like effect (not measurable) |
| **Hood** | 7-12 L/min | • Device should be run through a blender<br>• Ensure adequate flow to flush $CO_2$ from hood<br>• Noise from air flow is a concern - may lead to hearing impairment<br>• Incubator (Isolette) may be able to deliver O₂, but this is usually not used clinically (limits patient access, difficult to maintain specific O₂%) |
| **Heated Humidified High Flow Nasal Cannula (HHHFNC)** | 1-8 L/min | • Device should be run through a blender (unless flow generator has a built-in blender)<br>• Several models use a specialized nasal cannula to accomodate the higher flows<br>• Likely creates PEEP-like effect (may measure amount produced, but not effective amount delivered)<br>• Some evidence suggests N-CPAP being more effective than HFNC |
| **N-CPAP** | *See Chapter 4* | |

# ■ inhaled Nitric Oxide (iNO)

- The body produces nitric oxide (endogenous) which regulates vascular tone, relaxing vascular smooth muscle
- Inhaled nitric oxide (iNO) is a selective pulmonary vasodilator ($\downarrow$PAP), resulting in smooth muscle relaxation of the vessels around the lungs. This allows for more effective perfusion in well-ventilated lung regions (improves V/Q matching). iNO is broken down quickly and thus has little effect on systemic vessels (SVR).

### Indications

- <u>Term or near-term (> 34 weeks gestation) neonates</u>: Normally systemic vascular resistance (SVR) surpasses pulmonary vascular resistance (PVR) at birth. In some disorders, SVR does not surpass PVR after birth, resulting in a continued shunting of blood which causes hypoxemia. (see diagram, next page)
- <u>Pediatric/adult acute hypoxemic respiratory failure</u> (including ARDS). Note that this indication does not have FDA approval, and there is no substantial evidence currently to support a change in morbidity or mortality.

### Hazards

- **Methemoglobinemia** (Nitric Oxide [NO] reacts with oxyhemoglobin to form an abnormal hemoglobin called methemoglobin). Monitor methemoglobin levels within 4-8 hours after treatment initiation, and then periodically. If Methemoglobinemia is noted, decrease or discontinue NO administration.
- **Rebound Pulmonary Hypertension Syndrome**: Occurs following abrupt discontinuation, with hypoxemia, hypotension, bradycardia. If noted, restart iNO immediately.
- **Nitrogen Dioxide ($NO_2$)**: When NO combines with $O_2$, $NO_2$ forms which inflames and damages the lungs. $NO_2$ should be monitored continually (through the iNO delivery system).
- **Worsened heart failure**: Some patients with left ventricular dysfunction experience pulmonary edema, $\uparrow$ PCWP, hypotension, bardycardia, and cardiac arrest. Discontinue iNO when noted.

## Neonatal Hypoxic Respiratory Failure associated with Pulmonary Hypertension

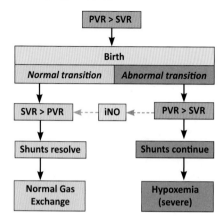

### Dosaging

Initiate therapy at 20 PPM. Maintain treatment for up to 14 days, or until underlying oxygen desaturation has resolved.

### Management and Weaning

- The goal is to aggressively wean $O_2\%$ once iNO is initiated.
- Once $O_2\%$ is at a safer range (and $PaO_2$ is at an acceptable range), weaning of iNO can begin.
- iNO should be weaned by cutting dose in half until at 5 ppm, then wean by 1 ppm until ready to discontinue. Assess carefully at each weaning step (return to previous step if unsuccessful). If oxygenation worsens at any point, go back up.

### Clinical Notes

- A slight decrease in oxygen concentration ($FIO_2$) occurs when adding iNO (800 ppm tank), which may result in $O_2\% < 21\%$ (at 20 PPM, with 21% $O_2$, the actual % delivered is ~20%).

- A slight change in delivered minute ventilation may occur due to the addition and removal of gases by the delivery system (+0.02 L/min at 20 ppm). Note that this has the potential to affect triggering.
- Circuits must be purged when not in use for any period of time due to accumulation of $NO_2$. Resuscitator bag should be squeezed several times to flush out $NO_2$ before connecting to a patient

## Inhaled Nitric Oxide Neonatal Management Algorithm

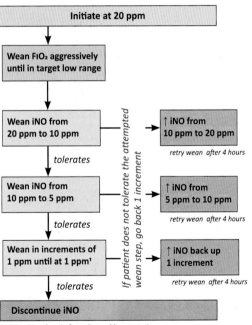

Monitor closely for rebound hypoxemia

[1]Some clinicians wean more rapidly, going from 5 ppm to 2 ppm, then discontinuing from there.

## Inhaled Nitric Oxide Duration Charts
## (800 ppm with INOMAX)[1]

**D-size cylinder**

| iNO dose (ppm) | Flow (L/min) | | | |
|---|---|---|---|---|
| | **5** | **10** | **20** | **40** |
| 5 | 7.0 days | 3.5 days | 1.8 days | 21 hours |
| 10 | 3.5 days | 1.7 days | 21 hours | 10.5 hours |
| 20 | 1.7 days | 20.7 hours | 10.3 hours | 5.2 hours |

**88-size cylinder**

| iNO dose (ppm) | Flow (L/min) | | | |
|---|---|---|---|---|
| | **5** | **10** | **20** | **40** |
| 5 | 39 days | 19.5 days | 9.8 days | 4.9 days |
| 10 | 19.4 days | 9.7 days | 4.8 days | 2.4 days |
| 20 | 9.6 days | 4.8 days | 2.4 days | 1.2 days |

[1]Tables based on manufacturer literature

## ■ Surfactant Administration

Neonatal

- Review AARC Clinical Practice Guideline (see next pages) for specific indications, strategies, contraindications, monitoring, hazards, delivery techniques
- See Pharmacology Chapter (pg 7-32 and following) for specific pharmacologic agents, dosing, dosing charts, and for specific administration recommendations (routes, positioning)

**Notes:**
- There is debate and variance in practice:
  - <u>Prophylactic administration</u>: due to presence of risk factors, particularly prematurity
  - <u>Rescue administration</u>: in the presence of confirmed need, such as clinical evidence of respiratory distress syndrome. *Once there is evidence of RDS, administration should not be delayed*
- Multiple-dose surfactant therapy is common, with ↓ mortality
- The bedside clinician should be acutely aware of ventilator parameters (or pressures when bagging), as these are likely to change rapidly upon surfactant administration (rapid ↑ in CL is expected). Note that this can have an adverse effect on an existent PDA, resulting in hemorrhage.
- Doses generally are given by a catheter (feeding tube) advanced through ET Tube (NOTE: ET tube position must be confirmed prior to administering), or via a sideport on the ET Tube. Specific manufacturer recommendations are in the pharmacology chapter, although current evidence supports administration through catheter or dual-lumen ET Tube.
- Doses are given in 2 or 4 aliquots. Specific manufacturer recommendations are in the pharmacology chapter, although current evidence supports keeping the patient supine, with chest horizontal.
- Suctioning should be avoided for 2 hours post-administration unless significant adverse effects are noted
- Adverse effects are noted in the AARC Clinical Practice Guideline (following pages), but are generally transient

## Surfactant Replacement Therapy[1]
### (AARC Clinical Practice Guideline)

**Description**

Surfactant is a compound that forms a layer between the alveolar surface and the alveolar gas and reduces alveolar collapse by decreasing surface tension within the alveoli. This improves lung compliance and stabilizes lung volumes at lower transpulmonary pressures

Surfactant may also enhance macrophages and mucociliary clearance, as well as reduce inflammation

Premature neonates are more likely to be surfactant-deficient.

**Two strategies:**

1. Prophylactic (at birth or after birth to infants at high risk of developing RDS
2. Rescue (after clinical confirmation of RDS)

**Indications**

Prophylactic administration:

High risk RDS (< 32 weeks gestation or < 1300 g)

Surfactant deficiency (laboratory evidence) L/S < 2:1

Bubble stability test

Absence of phosphatidylglycerol

Rescue/therapeutic administration:

Require intubation/ventilation due to respiratory failure, with an $FiO_2 \geq 0.40$ and evidence of RDS or MAS, including neonates with mPAW > 7 $cmH_2O$ to maintain adequate $O_2$

**Other Uses**

Delivery of other drugs (antibiotics, anti-inflammatory, bronchodilators)

Post-op development of ARDS following cardiac surgery

Treatment of severe RSV (porcine surfactant) may improve gas exchange

**Contraindications**

RDS in infants with mature lungs

Congenital abnormalities incompatible with life beyond the neonatal period

Presence of congenital diaphragmatic hernia

Substantial pulmonary hypoplasia (this has weak evidence)

Hemodynamic instability

Active pulmonary hemorrhage

## (Surfactant Therapy continued from previous page)

**Hazards**
ET Tube plugging
↑ Need for $O_2$ initially
Bradycardia (hypoxia)
Tachycardia (agitation)
Pharyngeal deposition
Administered to only one lung
Pulmonary hemorrhage
↑ necessity to treat PDA
↑ risk of retinopathy of pre-
maturity
Volutrauma

**Assessment of Outcome**
↓ in $FIO_2$ requirement
↓ WOB
Improved aeration on CXR
Improved pulmonary me-
chanics and lung volumes
Able to titrate ventilator set-
tings down
Improved P(A-a)$O_2$, OI

**Equipment/Resources**
Syringe of surfactant
Feeding tube/catheter, ET con-
necter with delivery port, or
closed catheter system
Ventilator with VT monitoring
Resuscitation equipment
Monitoring equipment (VT,
$SpO_2$, Cardiac)

**Monitoring**
Placement of delivery device
$FIO_2$, Vent setting
Reflux of surfactant
Patient position
Chest wall movement
$SpO_2$
Vital signs
Pulmonary mechanics, VT
Breath sounds

**Delivery Techniques**

INSURE
(*In*tubation, *Sur*factant,
*E*xtubation)
Surfactant is administered
early, then infant is promptly
extubated to N-CPAP

Administer on Vent (higher settings), then titrate ventilator
settings down and extubate.
Used with clinical indications
of RDS

Pharyngeal instillation before
first breath, then infant is
stimulated to breathe

Laryngeal Mask Airway
administration (when ET Tube
intubation skills are lacking)

Bronchoalveolar Lavage -
primarily for meconium
aspiration syndrome (MAS)

Adapted from AARC Clinical Practice Guideline, Respiratory Care,
Vol. 58 (2), 2013.

**Transport**

**CONTENTS**

## ▣ Indications

- Transport a neonate/child from lower- to higher-level facility
- Reverse Transport (higher-to-lower) is occasional—convalescence
- Major goal is to safely transport stabilized child

**American Academy of Pediatrics: Hospital Level Designations**

| | |
|---|---|
| **Level I** | • Resuscitate, evaluate and provide postnatal care of healthy newborn infants<br>• Care for 35-37 wk gestation who are physiologically stable<br>• Stabilize ill infants until transfer to a facility that can provide the appropriate level of neonatal care |
| **Level II** | Provide care to infants born > 32 wk gestation and weighing 1500+ grams at birth who have (are):<br><br>• Physiologic immaturity: apnea of prematurity, body temp issues, or inability to take oral feedings<br>• Moderately ill with problems likely to resolve rapidly and not likely to need urgent subspecialty services<br>• Convalescing from a higher level of intensive care<br>• Provide noninvasive (CPAP) or invasive ventilation for brief duration (< 24 hours) |
| **Level III** | Provide continuous life support and comprehensive care for extremely high-risk newborn infants and those with critical illness ( < 1500 g or at < 32 weeks' gestation)<br>• Provide critical medical and surgical care<br>• Provide ongoing assisted ventilation<br>• Ready-access to a full range of pediatric medical subspecialists<br>• Advanced imaging with interpretation<br>• Ready-access to pediatric ophthalmologists, pediatric surgical specialists and pediatric anesthesiologists |
| **Level IV** | Level III NICU AND can provide on-site surgical repair of serious congenital or acquired malformations<br>• Can facilitate transport / provide outreach educ. |

**Transfer to a higher level facility should be considered for any patient presenting care challenges unable to be met at the current level.**

This includes:

## Neonatal Conditions

- Gestation < 34 wks, Weight < 2,000 grams
- Respiratory distress (oxygenation or ventilation)
- Birth asphyxia or shock
- Congenital defects
- Meconium aspiration (below vocal cords, with distress)
- Cardiac disorders w/ persisting cyanosis
- Hypoglycemia (persistent)
- Hypovolemia (low BP and poor perfusion)
- Seizures

## Maternal Conditions:

### Obstetric
- Premature Rupture of Membranes (PROM)
- Premature labor
- Severe preeclampsia
- IUGR with fetal distress

### Medical
- Infections (may result in premature birth)
- Heart disease (Class III or IV)
- Drug overdose

### Surgical
- Trauma/surgery requiring intensive care
- Thoracic emergencies requiring intensive care or surgery

## Pediatric Conditions

- Depressed or deteriorating neurological status
- Children requiring ventilatory support beyond what referring facility is able to provide
- Need for ECMO (Pediatric ARDS, etc.)
- Shock—compensated or uncompensated
- Injuries requiring blood transfusion
- Significant trauma injuries (head injury, fracture of two or more major long bones, spinal cord injuries, traumatic amutation, wounds or blunt injury to chest/abdomen)

## student tip          Neonatal Transport

For many students (and new graduates), the idea of flying out to a remote facility and transporting an unstable neonate sounds pretty exciting (and it can be). How do you work towards this?

It is a combination of TRAINING and EXPERIENCE.

### Training:

Obviously working in a fast-paced, regional NICU with an exceptional mentor is a great way to get this training. Consider going through S.T.A.B.L.E. (see pg 6-6 for a summary), and volunteer to help with anything and everything in the NICU. In addition, there are some residency programs which mentor you into this important role.

### Experience:

Experience comes by, well, doing it. While safety is paramount, you must jump in and start doing things. Once on a transport you will hopefully be partnered with an exceptional medical professional (RN, etc.) but ultimately you are the respiratory expert! Becoming an expert means saturating yourself with information and applying it over and over.

Simulations are an exceptional opportunity to practice in a safe environment, as well!

## Transport Timeline

| Referring Team | |
|---|---|
| 1. Make Referral | Refer as quickly as possible to allow for transport team to travel and to receive coaching support |
| 2. Stabilization | STABLE (next page) Maternal (see pg 6-8) Neonatal (see pg 6-8) |
| Transport Team (higher level of care facility) | |
| 3. Prepare | Check equipment and supplies (pg 6-17) |
| (Transport Team Travels to the Referral Site) | Maintain good communication and coaching (as needed) with referring facility. |
| 4. Stabilize | See pg 6-19 |
| 5. Prepare for Departure | See pg 6-20 |
| 6. Just prior to Departure | See pg 6-21 |
| 7. Transport | See pg 6-21 |
| 8. Arrival at Higher Level Facility | See pg 6-21 |

Transport

# Overview of S.T.A.B.L.E program[1]
### *Pre-Transport / Post-Resuscitation Stabilization Care*

*What is STABLE? It is a program designed to provide a framework of care for community hospitals to stabilize a neonate until a transport team can arrive and take the infant to a facility with additional supports.*

*It starts after resuscitation, so assumes competence in neonatal resuscitation (NRP).*

| | |
|---|---|
| **S  Sugar & Safe Care**<br><br>See pg 6-13 | • Do not give oral or enteral feedings if sick (↑ risk of aspiration)<br>• Provide glucose by IV<br>• Neonates at ↑ risk include SGA, LGA, IDM, stressed, and certain maternal drugs<br>• **UVC if**: Rapid access diff. with peripheral access, > 1 IV line required, administration of > 12.5% dextrose indicated, or to perform exchange transfusion<br>• **UAC if**: Hemo monitoring (continuous BP), or frequent ABGs indicated |
| **T  Temperature**<br><br>See pg 6-10 | • Maintain *thermal neutral temperature* (36.5-37.5°C)<br>• Consider therapeutic hypothermia for Hypoxic-Ischemic Encephalopathy (HIE)<br>• COLD STRESS will cause:<br>  • vasoconstriction (periph + lungs)<br>  • ↑ muscle flexion/activity<br>  • Brown fat metabolism<br>*Younger Gestation Age may not be able to vasoconstrict, flex, and these neonates have ↓ brown fat supplies |
| **A  Airway**<br><br>SEE Ch 5 | • Identify neonatal distress and resp failure<br>• Provide airway management when necessary<br>• Consider non-pharmacologic strategies for managing pain (sucking, swaddling, tucking, kangaroo care, music therapy)<br>• Minor procedures: oral sucrose solution<br>• Stronger analgesia: morphine or fentanyl |

| | | |
|---|---|---|
| **B** | **Blood Pressure**<br><br>**SEE Ch 10 - SHOCK** | • Understand compensated shock (BP is maintained by shunting blood from non-vital organs but increases anaerobic metabolism [↑ acidosis]) versus uncompensated shock (hypotension present).<br>• Identify and treat typical shock: hypovolemic, cardiogenic, septic |
| **L** | **Lab Work** | • Identify and treat signs of infection EARLY (due to immaturity of immune system, consequences of infection can be severe)<br>• Signs/Symptoms of sepsis are variable. Treat aggressively (antibiotics) at first sign<br>• Labs **before** transport:<br>  • Blood Count (CBC with WBC diff and platelets)<br>  • Blood Culture (before antibiotics)<br>  • Blood Glucose (check early)<br>  • Blood Gas (when respiratory distress, shock, and/or infection are present)<br>• Labs **after** transport:<br>  • CSF (meningitis)<br>  • Electrolytes ($Na^+$, $K^+$)<br>  • Ionized calcium<br>  • BUN/Creatinine<br>  • Liver enzymes (AST, ALT, GGT)<br>  • Bilirubin (conjugated + unconjugated)<br>  • Coagulation studies<br>  • Magnesium (if administered to mom) |
| **E** | **Emotional Support** | • Support parent(s) during key stages:<br>  • Initial stabilization period<br>  • Arrival of transport team<br>  • After transport (initially and in NICU)<br>• Facilitate parenting in the NICU |

[1] This is a selected summary of the guidelines found in the S.T.A.B.L.E. program. Complete details on participating in the program can be found at stableprogram.org.

## ■ 1. Referral

While the referral process is beyond the scope of this book, the following is important to note:

- Referrals should be made in a timely manner (after resuscitation, but before stabilization)
- Pertinent neonatal <u>and</u> maternal data should be provided
- The family should be communicated with often regarding the process

## ■ 2. Stabilization *(see also Chapter 2)*

All hospitals need to ensure they can care for an unstable neonate/child for up to 4 hours (or beyond in rural areas).  See Transport (page 6-16 and following) for more discussion of considerations.

### Maternal Stabilization

- Provide hemodynamic support
- Initiate tocolytics, anticonvulsants or antihypertensive agents as indicated (see pg 2-15)
- May initiate antibiotics and/or betamethasone for appropriate patients with consultation from receiving hospital
- Initiate treatment for active bleeding, preeclampsia, or rapidly progressive labor
- The possibility of delivery or the development of an acute crisis in transport should be minimized
- If maternal transport is not advisable, the transport team could consider traveling to the delivery to assist in initial stabilization

### Neonatal Stabilization

**Priorities** *(see following pages for details)*

| Goal | to Prevent/Correct |
|---|---|
| **A. Respiratory Support** | Asphyxia, Hypoxia, Hypercarbia |
| **B. Thermal Support** | Hypothermia, unless therapeutic |
| **C. Hemodynamic Support** | Hypovolemia, Hypotension |
| **D. Glucose Homeostasis** | Hypoglycemia |
| **E. Acid-Base Balance** | Acidosis |
| **F. Other Supports** | UO/X-Ray/Gastric |

## A. Respiratory Support

| | |
|---|---|
| **Airway** | Ensure open airway<br>Suction as needed (*max* 80-100 mmHg) |
| **Oxygenation** | Indications (see page 5-15)<br>Keep PaO$_2$ 50-80 mmHg or give just enough to relieve central cyanosis if no ABGs available<br>Keep O$_2$ Sat > 85%<br>O$_2$ should be delivered as accurately as possible (blender or venturi)<br>A hood inside an incubator is better than flooding the incubator<br>The FiO$_2$ should be analyzed continuously<br>Warm & humidify gases (cause hypothermia)<br>Use CPAP if indicated (pg 4-20) & available (do not use in CDH or other air-trapping illnesses) |
| **Ventilation** | Keep PaCO$_2$ 40-55 mmHg (permissive hypercapnia now widely used)<br>Manual ventilation — <u>always</u> use with a pressure manometer in line & keep PIP as low as possible to still achieve adequate chest expansion and breath sounds<br>Indications for intubation and mech. vent. (see pgs 5-5, 4-5)<br>Do not use ventilators unless designed for neonatal/pediatric use<br>Prefer bag-mask ventilation to misplaced ET Tube. If in doubt: extubate and BVM ventilate. |

**Target Blood Gas Values**

| | < 28 wk EGA | 28-40 wk EGA | Term with PPHN | Term with BPD |
|---|---|---|---|---|
| **PaO$_2$** | 45-65 | 50-70 | 80-120 | 50-80 |
| **PaCO$_2$** | 45-55 | 45-60 | 30-40 | 55-65 |
| **pH** | $\geq 7.25$ | > 7.25 | 7.30-7.50 | 7.35-7.47 |

Adapted from: Durand DJ et al. Blood gases: Technical aspects and interpretation, Goldsmith JP. Assisted ventilation of the neonate. 4th Ed., Saunders, 2003: 279-292

| **B. Thermal Support** | |
|---|---|
| Support | Immediately place in neutral thermal environment |
| | Use warmer, double wall incubator, plastic heat shield, or plastic blankets as indicated and available. |
| | Very Low Birth Weight (VLBW): consider wrapping body (not head) in plastic wrap to prevent insensible water loss |
| | Only use warm water bottles if no other options, and avoid direct skin contact |
| | Do not use gooseneck lamps (burn hazard) |
| | Minimize time outside incubator |
| | Use portals only for manipulation |
| | Keep abdominal skin temp 36—36.5°C |
| | Correct hypothermia — to heat up, use an environmental temp of max 1.5° C > abdominal temperature |
| | Avoid keeping baby in cold environment such as delivery room where temps may be 60-65° — this will undermine attempts to thermoregulate |
| | Normal core temp: 36.5-37.5° C |
| | Maintain body temp of 37° C. Monitor every 15-30 mins until within normal range, then every hour |

**Hypothermia** *(per World Health Org.)*

| Mild | 36-36.4° C |
|---|---|
| Moderate | 32-35.9° C |
| Severe | < 32° C |

| Signs and Symptoms of Hypothermia | Hypoxia |
|---|---|
| | ↓ peripheral perfusion |
| | ↑ PVR |
| | Hypoglycemia |
| | Metabolic acidosis |

| Therapeutic Hypothermia | Management of Hypoxic-Ischemic Encephalopathy (HIE) |
|---|---|

**Criteria** (ALL must be met):
1. Gestational age $\geq$ 35 weeks
2. Birth weight $\geq$ 1800 grams
3. $\leq$ 6 hours since insult has occurred[1].

**If all 3 criteria above are met then at least 1 of the following must also be met:**
1. pH $\geq$ 7.0 with base deficit $\geq$ 16 by an ABG
2. pH 7.01-7.15 with base deficit 10-15.9 or no ABG available an acute perinatal event (cord prolapse, HR decelerations, uterine rupture, etc.) and EITHER:
   - APGAR $\leq$ 5 at 10 minutes OR
   - Assisted Ventilation $\geq$ 10 mins with seizures

**Contraindications**:
- Suspected or presence of lethal chromosomal abnormalities
- Severe intrauterine growth restriction (IUGR)
- Significant intracranial hemorrhage[2] (Grade III or Grade IV)

**Procedure**: Cool infant down to a temperature of 33.5 C (92.3 F) for 72 hours.

*Referring Facility*:
- Passive Cooling: turn radiant warmer off, monitor core temp every 15 min with goal of 33.5° C
- If temp drops < 33.0° C, turn on radiant warmer (set temp 0.5° C above current temp)
- Increase by 0.5° C every 30 mins until at 33.5° C, then discontinue

[1] Studies show that the initiation of cooling within 6 hrs of birth has ↓ the incidence of death and severe disability in neonates with HIE
[2] If ultrasound is not immediately available, start cooling process and follow up with ultrasound confirmation as soon as able

| C. Hemodynamic Support | |
|---|---|
| **Maintain Pulse** | Maintain HR > 120/min |
| **Maintain Systolic BP** | **Maintain systolic BP:** Ex: > 40 mmHg (l Kg)<br>(rough guidelines) > 50 mmHg (2 Kg)<br> > 60 mmHg (3 Kg)<br><br>BPsys = (wt[Kg] + 3)10<br>**MAP should be at least equal to gestational age** |
| **Maintain Hematocrit** | Maintain hematocrit > 40%<br><br>*if anemic:* Begin cross-match procedure before transport for emergency: use non-cross matched type O neg cells |
| **Correct Hypovolemia** | 10 cc/kg normal saline<br>*(may need 20-300 cc's for true hypovolemia)* |
| **Signs and Symptoms of Hypovolemia** | • Persistent ↑ in heart rate<br>• Skin gray, dusky, pale and cool<br>• ↓ capillary refill<br>• ↓ BP<br>• Weak femoral pulses<br>• ↓ CVP (via UVC)<br>• ↓ Urine Output (< 1 mg/Kg/hr) |
| **Vascular Access** | • Peripheral IV may be adequate<br>• A-Line and/or CVP preferred<br>• UAC - used most often<br>• UVC - quickest and easiest |

| Line Placement | High | Low |
|---|---|---|
| **UAC** | T6-T8 | L3-L4 |
| **UVC** | T11-T12<br>(above diaphragm, not in heart) | Should be placed high |

| D. Glucose Homeostasis | |
|---|---|
| **Support** | **Maintain plasma glucose ~40-110 mg/dL[1]**<br>**Glucose Management[2]:**<br>Symptomatic:<br> < 48 hrs old + plasma glucose < 50 mg/dL<br> > 48 hrs old + plasma glucose < 60 mg/dL<br>Asymptomatic but at risk:<br> < 4 hrs old + plasma glucose < 25 mg/dL<br> 4-24 hrs old + plasma glucose < 35 mg/dL<br> 24-48 hrs old + plasma glucose < 50 mg/dL<br> > 48 hrs old + plasma glucose < 60 mg/dL |

| Daily Fluid Requirements →→ (mL/kg/day) | 60 | 80 | 100 |
|---|---|---|---|
| $D_{10}W$ (mg/kg/min) | 4.2 | 5.5 | 6.9 |
| $D_{12.5}W$ (mg/kg/min) | 5.2 | 6.9 | 8.7 |
| $D_{15}W$ (mg/kg/min) | 6.3 | 8.3 | 10.4 |

*< 34 wks gest:* IV 1-2 **mL**/kg/dose D10W
then cont. IV 4-6 **mg**/kg/min
*> 34 wks gest:* IV 2 **mL**/kg/dose D10W
+/or cont. IV 5-8 **mg**/kg/min titrated
to maintain ≥ 40-50 mg/dL
*More than $D_{15}W$ requires central line*

| Signs and Symptoms of Hypoglycemia | Apnea/Bradycardia<br>Cyanosis<br>Hypotonia<br>LOC changes<br>Hypothermia | Tachypnea<br>Tremors/Jitters<br>Poor suck/feeding<br>Seizures |
|---|---|---|

| Significant Risk Factors for Hypoglycemia | **Premie**<br> SGA<br> LGA<br> RDS<br> Asphyxia | **Stressed**<br> IDM<br> Sepsis<br> Hypothermic<br> Polycythemia |
|---|---|---|

[1] STABLE recommends a range of 50-110 mg/dL
[2] Per *2011 Amer. Acad. of Pediatrics (AAP)*

| E. Acid-Base Balance | |
|---|---|
| **Respiratory Acidosis** | Correct alveolar ventilation<br>   Noninvasive (often the preferred choice)<br>   Invasive |
| **Metabolic Acidosis** | **Correct oxygenation, ventilation, and perfusion, then:**<br><u>If persistent, give NaHCO₃ therapy when[1]:</u><br>  • pH < 7.20<br>  • $HCO_3$ < 15 mEq/L *and*<br>  • Base Deficit > 10 mEq/L<br><br>(mEq $NaHCO_3$ = BD × 0.3 × Kg)<br>(infuse < 1 mL/Kg/min)<br><br>[1] controversial |

| F. Other Supports | |
|---|---|
| **Urine Output** | Normal UO = 1-2 mL/kg/hr<br>Place Urine Bag on all transports |
| **X-Ray Indications** | **Chest:**<br>  Respiratory Distress or lung pathology<br>  CHF<br>  Diaphragmatic hernia<br>  Esophageal atresia or T-E Fistula<br>**Abdomen:** Distention<br>**Tubes/Catheters:** Verify location |
| **NG/OG Tubes** | All patients should have stomach contents aspirated prior to transport<br>Tube may be left in or removed, as indicated<br><br>**Absolute Indications:**<br>  • Diaphragmatic hernia<br>  • Ventilation with Bag/Mask<br>  • N-CPAP<br>  • Bowel Obstruction or Ileus<br>  • E-A or T-E Fistula<br>  • Vomiting |

# Pediatric Stabilization

The transport environment is a relatively unstable environment for performing procedures. Preventive measures are often preferable to reactive ones.

It is critical to avoid transporting an unstable child. The referring team and receiving team should work together to ensure the child is as stable as possible **before transport begins, including:**

- **Securing the Airway—consider:**
  - Child age/size
  - Trend in patient condition (towards more stable or less stable)
  - Comorbidities
  - Behavior (anxiety, combativeness, etc.)
  - Sedative/analgesic needs (burns, etc.)
- Ensure ET tube cuff is not overinflated
- Any trapped air (pneumothorax, etc.) should be considered before air transport in an unpressurized aircraft, as gas volume will increase at altitude. Consider draining even small pneumothoraces.
- Perform thorough assessment prior to transport. Auscultation may be difficult or impossible, motion artifact may play a disruptive role in $SpO_2$ and BP.
- If intubated, ensure adequate sedation to avoid potential for inadvertent extubation
- Ensure adequate body temperature as small children lose significant heat through radiant/evaporative/conductive transfer
  - Hypothermia increases myocardial stress
  - Fever should be avoided with cardiac arrest and brain injury
- Ensure adequate supplies and equipment for pediatric patients (see next section)

# ■ Transport (Transport Team)

**Factors to Consider in Selecting Transport Mode**
- **Travel Time** (optimal goal = < 2 hours one-way)
- **Weather**
- Landing sites (air)/need for ground transport on landing
- Two-way communication available (cell or satellite phone)
- Noise, vibration, rotation
- Pressurization of aircraft (fixed wing - maybe, helicopters - no)
- **Appropriate equipment**: Oxygen, Air, Suction
- Cabin temp needs to be monitored/controlled: air or ground
- **Be aware of voltage differences** in various transport modes

## Modes of Transport
*(green = strengths, yellow = variable, red = limitation)*

| Factor | Ground | Rotary[1] | Fixed-Wing |
|---|---|---|---|
| Distance[2] | < 25 miles | < 150 miles | > 150 miles |
| Noise | Varies | | |
| Altitude Effects (oxygenation) | | not usually pressurized | pressurized to ~2500m |
| Temp (environment) ↓ 2°C/300m altitude | | | |
| Cost | | | |
| Time to Departure | | | |
| Time to Arrival | | | |
| Weather Issues | | | |
| Access to Patient | | | |
| Speed | | | |
| Space (landing, etc.) | | | |

[1] Rotary = helicopter
[2] Distance factors are overridden at times by weather (for example, ground transport may be the only option if weather is poor)

### 3. Prepare (check supplies and equipment)

**Gas Supply (Air, $O_2$):** Check pressures (Carry 2X the calculated $O_2$ requirement), see the chart on next page

**Necessary wrenches/adaptors:** Equipment/Gas connections

**Remember:** There are too many quick-connects to carry all possible options, so prepare ahead with tanks or call ahead

**$O_2$ supply required** for MVs. Requires dialed-in flowrate + flowrate required to run vent (see vent specs in manuals)

**Transport Ventilator, tanks, etc.** should be checked on transport stretcher/isolette

**Confirm battery life/elec. equipment function and calibration**

**Transport Bag:** Ensure all equipment possibly needed is packed; consider rechecking, even if tagged. Include:

#### Essential Equipment in Respiratory Transport Bag

|  |  |
|---|---|
|  | Ventilator circuits (extra) |
|  | Heater probes (extra) |
|  | Humidifier |
|  | Oxygen analyzer and t-piece |
|  | Bag/Mask (neonatal, infant)<br> - a self-inflating BVM should always be packed<br>   (in case of gas failure) |
|  | Airway equipment:<br>  ET Tubes<br>  LMA (appropriate sizes for age)<br>  Laryngoscopes/Blades + extra batteries/bulbs<br>    (include #1 Mac blade - see Pierre-Robin)<br>  $ETCO_2$ (continuous or colorimetric)<br>  Suction catheters<br>  Suction tubing + canister<br>  Stethoscope |
|  | Neo/Infant: Nasal prongs (various sizes) for N-CPAP |
|  | Oxygen delivery equipment (several sizes) |

**Estimated Cylinder Duration**

| | Flow | 2000 PSI | 1500 PSI | 1000 PSI | 500 PSI |
|---|---|---|---|---|---|
| **E cylinder MINUTES** | 2 | 280 | 210 | 140 | 70 |
| | 4 | 140 | 105 | 70 | 35 |
| | 10 | 56 | 42 | 28 | 14 |
| | 15 | 37 | 28 | 19 | 9 |
| **H cylinder HOURS** | 2 | 52 | 39 | 26 | 13 |
| | 4 | 26 | 19 | 13 | 6 |
| | 10 | 10 | 7 | 5 | 2 |
| | 15 | 6 | 5 | 3 | 1 |

**To Calculate Cylinder Flow Time (Duration)**

1. Conversion Factor = $\dfrac{\text{cylinder volume (in cu. ft.) X 28.3}}{\text{Max } P_{cyl}}$
   (or chart below)

2. Cylinder Flow Time (minutes) = $\dfrac{\text{Cyl Pressure (Pcyl) X CF}}{\text{Flowrate}}$

| Cylinder Conversion Factors (CF) | | |
|---|---|---|
| **Size** | **cu. ft.** | **factor** |
| A | 2.7 | 0.035 |
| B | 5.3 | 0.068 |
| D | 12.6 | 0.16 |
| E | 22 | 0.28 |
| G | 186 | 2.41 |
| H/K | 244 | 3.14 |
| M | 128 | 1.65 |

## 4. Stabilize

Complete any stabilization procedures not accomplished by the referring hospital. (The team should remember that the referring hospital personnel have probably performed to the best of their ability, regardless of pt's condition). Each visit should present as a teaching and learning opportunity.

*Stabilization prior to transport is probably the most important aspect of inter-hospital care. Patient deterioration enroute may not be detectable or as easily treatable.*

Stabilize as completely as feasible the following:
Temp, ABGs ($O_2$, vent, pH), vascular volume, vitals, and glucose
Complete stabilization may not be possible but transport of an extremely unstable infant is usually contraindicated unless pt cannot be stabilized at referring hospital.
If transporting on prostaglandins it is important to have a 2nd IV in case the first one is lost.

| Evaluate: | Apply/Initiate: | Assess: |
|---|---|---|
| • History | • Vital monitoring | • Primary diagnosis |
| • Physical exam | • $FIO_2$ analysis | • Patient's condition |
| • ABGs | • IV access | • Complicating |
| • X-Rays | | conditions |
| • Labs | | |

**See Disease and Disorder Chapter for transport considerations of specific diseases and disorders.**

## 5. Prepare for Departure

**Intubate** — if clinically indicated and/or any possibility of needing enroute: definitely is advisable if by helicopter. (e.g., PGE infusion-related apnea) (CXR to confirm position).

### Estimated Tube Size (Neonatal)

| Tube Size (I.D.) | Pt Weight | Gest Age |
|---|---|---|
| 2.5 mm | < 1000 gm | < 28 wks |
| 3.0 mm | 1000-2000 gm | 28-34 wks |
| 3.5 mm | 2000 - 3000 gm | 34-38 wks |
| 3.5 - 4.0 mm | > 3000 gm | > 38 wks |

**Depth of Intubation:** 6 cm + weight (kg)

ET tube positioning:  1000 gm - 7 cm @ lip
2000 gm - 8 cm @ lip
3000 gm - 9 cm @ lip
Ensure ET tube is well secured.

| 1-2-3-4 Rule | |
|---|---|
| 1 x ETT size = | ETT Size |
| 2 x ETT size = | NG, Foley, Sx cath size |
| 3 x ETT size = | ETT depth |
| 4 x ETT size = | Chest-tube size |

<u>Remember:</u>  Stabilizing baby while in a stable environment is much preferred over attempting to stabilize en route

- Initiate Mechanical Ventilation (transport vent) if any possibility of needing it enroute
- Mechanical ventilation is preferred over manual ventilation
- **Self-inflating bags** do not need air source and have pop-off valves which may be safer and more consistent than flow-inflating bags. **A pressure manometer is <u>always</u> used.**
- Chest tube placement (or Heimlich valve) - insert before transport. Trapped Gas expansion may occur via air transport.
- Ensure transport incubator is warm; begin heating when leaving for referring hospital.

## 6. Just Prior to Departure

Ensure adequate gas supply
Ensure ventilator is properly adjusted
Obtain all docs & specimens (lab, x-ray, mom & cord blood, etc.)
Call and give brief report to receiving hospital

**Visit parents**
Let parents see and touch child, if possible, and leave photo of
child with the family, provide emotional support

## 7. Transport (en Route)

**Continuous monitoring (or checks every 15 min) should include:**

| Infant | Temperature | Activity |
|---|---|---|
| | HR & EKG | IV Therapy |
| | RR & pattern | $O_2$ Sat |
| | BP | Blood glucose |
| | Color | (Chemstrip®) |
| **Ventilator** | Parameters | PEEP |
| | PIP or $V_T$ | Gas pressures |
| | Rate | |
| **Maternal** | HR | Cervical dilation |
| | RR & pattern | Fetal HR |
| | BP | Deep tendon reflexes |
| | Uterine contractions | IV therapy |

- Consider alternative referral sites or temporary stops in case
of vehicle malfunction or patient deterioration

- Consider and assign team roles in emergency situations

- Schedule regular mock drills to ensure and reinforce role
effectiveness

## 8. Upon Arrival

- Assist with admission as indicated
- Call back referring hospital to notify of safe arrival
- Complete documentation and clearly communicate to staff
- Immediately restock transport supplies
- Evaluate transport and debrief on any events

| **Physiological effects of altitude (non-pressurized aircraft)** | |
|---|---|
| ✈ **↑ Altitude** | $\downarrow P_IO_2 \rightarrow \downarrow P_aO_2 \rightarrow \uparrow PDA$ <br><br> **Action:** $\uparrow F_IO_2$ <br> **Adjusted $F_IO_2$ =** <br> $(F_IO_2 \times PB1 / PB2)$ <br> PB1= Initial baro press on ground <br> PB2 = current alt pressure (in air) |
| | **Gas expansion (closed spaces)** <br><br> Thoracic gas → air leaks <br> Intestinal gas → <br> distention → <br> ↑ diaph, vomit, aspiration <br> Ensure NG tube is placed in <br> <u>all</u> air transport patients <br> Air space above IV bottle <br> ↑ pressure → <br> forcible infusion <br> Keep vent port open. Use <br> infusion pump or vacuum <br> packed infusion bags. |
| ✖ **↓ Altitude** | $\uparrow P_IO_2 \rightarrow \uparrow P_aO_2 \rightarrow \uparrow FVP^1$ <br><br> **Action:** Adjust $F_IO_2$ accordingly <br> *(particularly on descent after titrating $O_2$ up during a flight)* |
| | **Gas contraction** <br> Air space above IV bottle <br> ↓ pressure → <br> vacuum → <br> hemorrhage <br> into IV line (see above) |

$^1$ FVP = fibrovascular proliferation (growth of abnormal vessels in the eyes), which may ↑ risk of Retinopathy of Prematurity.

## Altitude Chart

| Altitude (ft) | Barometric Pressure (mmHg) | FiO₂ Required to Maintain Constant PaO₂ [1] | | | | | | | | | PiO₂ While Breathing: | | | | | Gas Volume Expansion (% at Sea Level) |
|---|---|---|---|---|---|---|---|---|---|---|---|---|---|---|---|---|
| | | | | | | | | | | | 0.21 | 0.40 | 0.60 | 0.80 | 1.0 | |
| 16000 | 412 | 0.41 | 0.59 | 0.78 | 0.98 | | | | | | 76 | 146 | 219 | 292 | 365 | 184 |
| 14000 | 446 | 0.37 | 0.53 | 0.71 | 0.89 | | | | | | 83 | 160 | 239 | 319 | 399 | 170 |
| 12000 | 483 | 0.34 | 0.49 | 0.65 | 0.81 | 0.98 | | | | | 91 | 174 | 262 | 349 | 436 | 157 |
| 10000 | 523 | 0.31 | 0.45 | 0.60 | 0.75 | 0.90 | | | | | 100 | 190 | 286 | 381 | 476 | 145 |
| 8000 | 564 | 0.29 | 0.41 | 0.55 | 0.69 | 0.83 | 0.96 | | | | 108 | 207 | 310 | 414 | 517 | 135 |
| 6000 | 609 | 0.27 | 0.38 | 0.51 | 0.63 | 0.76 | 0.89 | | | | 118 | 226 | 337 | 450 | 562 | 125 |
| 4000 | 656 | 0.24 | 0.35 | 0.47 | 0.58 | 0.70 | 0.82 | 0.94 | | | 127 | 244 | 365 | 487 | 609 | 116 |
| 2000 | 707 | 0.23 | 0.32 | 0.43 | 0.54 | 0.65 | 0.76 | 0.86 | 0.97 | | 138 | 264 | 396 | 528 | 660 | 107 |
| Sea Level | 760 | 0.21 | 0.30 | 0.40 | 0.50 | 0.60 | 0.70 | 0.80 | 0.90 | 1.0 | 149 | 285 | 428 | 570 | 713 | 100 |

1) As compared to that required at sea level.

$PIO_2 = (P_{B}-47)(FIO_2)$

$PAO_2 = PIO_2 - PaCO_2 (1.25)$

## CONTENTS

Always check manufacturers' inserts for changes in drug information to include dosages, indications, warnings, precautions and contraindications.

This chapter is not all-inclusive, but highlights drugs that directly affect respiratory care of neonatal and pediatric patients. Inhaled gases are covered in the respective procedures chapters.

## Abbreviations Used in Prescriptions

| | | | | | | |
|---|---|---|---|---|---|---|
| ā | before | IM | intra-muscular | q3h | every 3 hours |
| ac | before meals | IV | intra-vascular | q4h | every 4 hours |
| ad | to, up to | I&O | intake & output | qs, QS | as much as required |
| ad lib | as much as needed | L | liter/left | qt | quart |
| aq dist | distilled $H_2O$ | mixt | mixture | Rx | take |
| BID | 2x/day | mL | milliliter | s̄ | without |
| c̄ | with | NPO | nothing by mouth | sol | solution |
| caps | capsule | p̄ | after | solv | dissolve |
| dil | dilute | part acq | equal parts | SQ | subcutaneous |
| el, elix | elixir | pc | after meals | stat | immediately |
| emuls | emulsion | po | by mouth | syr | syrup |
| et | and | prn | as needed | tab | tablet(s) |
| ext | extract | rect | rectally | tid | 3x/day |
| fl, fld | fluid | pulv | powder | tinct | tincture |
| g, gm | gram | q | every | ung | ointment |
| gr | grain | qh | every hour | | |
| gtt | drop/drip | qid | 4x/day | | |
| hs | hour of sleep | q2h | every 2 hours | | |

# Adjusting for Pediatric Dosages

Remember that recommended dosages are only estimates. Dosages should be individualized - adjust for variations in maturity, metabolism, temperature, obesity, edema, illness, and individual tolerances.

Current literature supports BSA as the most consistent and accurate method of drug dosing over a wide range of body sizes. However, for small children (< 10 kg) dosing should be made on a mg/kg basis as BSA increases disproportionately as weight decreases.

Most drugs are dosed on a mg/kg basis in children. Due to variations in distribution, metabolism, and elimination, children require a higher mg/kg dose than adults. While this works well for younger children, in older larger children and adolescents (>40 kg), when dosed by this method, adult doses can often be exceeded.

For this reason:
**Never give a child a dose greater than the usual adult dose, regardless of height or weight.**

**Body Surface Area (Clark's BSA) Rule**

Estimated child's dose = $\dfrac{\text{Child's BSA (m}^2\text{) x Adult dose}}{1.73}$

BSA (m²) = $\sqrt{\dfrac{\text{height(cm) x weight(kg)}}{3600}}$

*Lamb, TK, Leung, D. More on Simplified Calculation of Body Surface Area. New England Journal of Medicine 1988: 318:1130*

**Estimation of BSA for Children of "Normal Height and Weight"**

| Weight | | Approximate Age | Surface Area (sq m) |
|--------|--------|-----------------|---------------------|
| kg | lb | | |
| 3 | 6.6 | Newborn | 0.2 |
| 6 | 13.2 | 3 months | 0.3 |
| 10 | 22 | 1 year | 0.45 |
| 20 | 44 | 5.5 years | 0.8 |
| 30 | 66 | 9 years | 1 |
| 40 | 88 | 12 years | 1.3 |
| 50 | 110 | 14 years | 1.5 |
| 65 | 143 | Adult | 1.7 |

*adapted from West's nomogram*

**Body Weight Rules**

Clark's Rule (patients > 2 yrs)

Child's dose = $\dfrac{\text{Body Wt (lbs) x adult dose}}{150}$

Weight-Based Dosing:

Dose = pediatric dose/kg x child's weight (kg)

**Age Rules (less accurate than BSA or weight-based)**

Fried's Rule (infants up to 2 yrs)

Infant's dose = $\dfrac{\text{age (mos) x adult dose}}{150}$

Young's Rule (2-12 yrs)

Child's dose = $\dfrac{\text{age (yrs) x adult dose}}{\text{age (yrs) + 12}}$

## Maternal Interventions to Delay Labor

| Class of Drug | Typical Drugs | Rationale |
|---|---|---|
| **Hormone** | Progesterone (vaginally) | Prophylactic, high risk patients, helps mature lungs |
| **Antenatal Corticosteroids** | Dexamethasone Betamethasone | Matures Lung<br><br>*Repeated doses may cause neonate to be smaller, but growth catches up over time* |
| **Antibiotics** | various | Useful with PPROM |
| **Tocolytic Drugs** *(suppress premature labor to allow baby to more fully mature)* | | |
| **Beta-Adrenergic Agonists** | Terbutaline IV | Relaxes smooth muscle |
| **Electrolyte** | Magnesium Sulfate | Decreases contractility by interfering with calcium<br><br>*Neonates may show signs of magnesium toxicity (respiratory and/or neuromuscular depression)* |
| **Calcium Channel Blockers** | Nifedipine (off label use) | Relaxes smooth muscle by inhibiting the influx and release of calcium |
| **COX Inhibitor** | Indomethacin | Relaxes smooth muscle by inhibiting release of calcium |

PPROM = Preterm Premature Rupture of the Membranes

## ■ Maternal Interventions to Advance Labor

| Class of Drug | Typical Drugs | Rationale |
|---|---|---|
| **Synthetic Prostaglandin** | Misoprostol (oral or vaginally) | **Off label Use** Causes uterine contractions and cervical thinning<br><br>May be used with Oxytocin |
| **Natural Prostaglandin** | Dinoprostone (Cervidil) (Prostin E2) | Causes uterine contractions and cervical thinning |
| **Hormone Neuropeptide** | Oxytocin Pitocin | Causes uterine contractions. May cause contractions to be stronger and delivery to be quicker than natural labor.<br><br>*May cause distress in the neonate - monitor closely.*<br><br>Cervix needs to be "ripe" to be effective. |

| Non-Pharmacological Interventions | |
|---|---|
| **Balloon Catheter** | Narrow tube with a small balloon is inserted into cervix and then inflated. It is left in place until the cervix has opened enough for the balloon to fall out on its own (~3 cm) |
| **Stripping Membranes (membrane sweeping)** | Stripping of the amniotic membrane from the uterus may trigger the release of prostaglandins (which help trigger labor). Procedure: a clinician puts a finger through the cervix and then sweeps it around the inside edge of the opening. |
| **Amniotomy** | Once cervix has started to dilate, and head is descended, a sterile device is inserted into vagina, and the amniotic sac gently ruptured. |

## Bronchodilators

### Adrenoreceptor Responses

| Receptor | Target |
|----------|--------|
| alpha-1 | Dilates pupils, contracts smooth muscle |
| beta-1 | Stimulates force/rate of heart |
| beta-2 | Bronchodilator of lungs, causes involuntary muscle tremors |

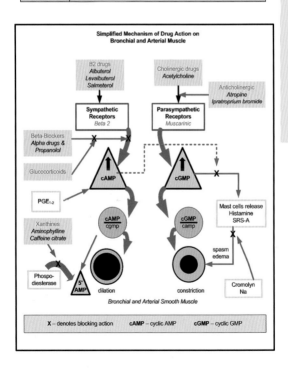

Simplified Mechanism of Drug Action on
Bronchial and Arterial Muscle

Bronchial and Arterial Smooth Muscle

X – denotes blocking action     cAMP – cyclic AMP     cGMP – cyclic GMP

# Assessing Response to Bronchodilator Therapy[1]

## Indications

**Assessment of airflow and other clinical indicators to:**
Confirm therapy is approp.
Individualized medication dose &/or frequency
Determine patient status during therapy
Determine need for changes in therapy (dose, frequency, types of medication)

## Contraindications

Some assessment maneuvers should be postponed during acute, severe distress.

## Hazards/Complications

Airway collapse
Bronchoconstriction
Coughing &/or syncope

## Frequency

**Acute, unstable patient –**
*Pre-therapy*: ABGs, full assessment, baseline values
*Pre and Post therapy*: BS, side effects, vital signs, PEFR, or FEV₁ (freq. is based upon acuteness and severity).
*Continuous*: SpO2

**Stable patient-**
*Hospital*: PEFR (pre and post therapy initially, then 2 x/ day.
*Home*: PEF initially 3-4x/day than 2x/day, depending on severity of symptoms.

## Assessment of Outcome/ Monitoring

**Pre-therapy (identify):**
Clinical indications
Contraindications
Respiratory and CV baseline values

**During therapy (identify):**
Adverse responses
Clinical changes

**Post therapy (identify):**
Adverse responses
Therapeutic responses
Lack of therapeutic responses

**Trend analysis (identify):**
Change in baseline
Need to – change therapy, discontinue therapy, modify dose

## Document

Patient responses and progress: breath sounds, lung function (PEFR, FEV, FVC), vital signs, symptoms.

**continued next page**

## Bronchodilator Therapy (continued)

| Monitoring | PFT's: |
|---|---|
| **Patient observation:** | FEV₁ &/or FVC (improved by 12% increase and 200mL increase) &/or FEF 25-75% improved, ↑PEF. |
| Accessory muscle use decreased | |
| General appearance improved | SaO₂, SpO₂ &/or ABG's improved |
| Sputum expectoration increased | Exercise performance improved |
| **Auscultation:** | Ventilator variables improved: |
| BS improved and volume of air moved is increased | Decreased: auto- PEEP, PIP, Pplat, Raw |
| Vital signs improved | Increased: expiratory flow |
| Subjective patient improvement | |

1) Adapted from AARC Clinical Practice Guidelines: Assessing Response to Bronchodilator Therapy at Point of Care, *Respiratory Care*, Volume 40, # 12, 1995.

## Bronchodilators: Summary of General Side Effects

| Pulmonary | Cardiovascular | CNS | Other |
|---|---|---|---|
| Bronchial irritation Bronchial edema | ↑BP, ↑HR, anginal pain, coronary insufficiency, palpitations, peripheral vasoconstriction | Anxiety/fear, headache, irritability, insomnia, restlessness, tremor, vertigo, weakness | Hypersensitivity, reaction to MDI propellants, tachyphylaxis, urinary retention, vomiting, nausea |

### Black Box Warning for LABAs *(see inserts for full warning)*

May increase the risk of asthma-related deaths. Use as a treatment for asthma not controlled with a control drug (such as an inhaled corticosteroid). Discontinue LABA as soon as possible after asthma control is attained. Consider use of combination products (e.g. LABA + Corticosteroid).

# Pharmacology

## Anti-Asthma - Mast Cell Stabilizers

| Medication | Dosage | Indications/Actions | Contraindications/Notes |
|---|---|---|---|
| cromolyn Na  *Nalcrom* | **INHALED SOLUTION:** 20 mg in 2 mL  **2 yr - adult:** 20 mg 4x/day may ↓ to 2-3x/day when stable  **ALLERGEN OR EIB:** Administer single dose 10-15 min, but not > 60 min, before precipitating event.  *SABA is more effective for EIA* | - Prophylactic mainte-nance of mild-to-moderate asthma - Not for acute exacerbations - Not as effective as SABA for Exercise-Induced Bronchoconstriction (EIB)  *Prevents release of inflammatory mediators from inflammatory cell types.* | **Adverse:** Bronchospasm, cough, local irritation, dry mouth, chest tightness, vertigo, unpleasant taste in mouth.  Neb solution (may dilute) may be mixed with albuterol.  Must be used at regular intervals for 2-4 weeks to be effective  Note that inhaled steroids are preferred for persistent asthma; cromolyn is an alternative option |

# Anti-asthma - Anti-Leukotrienes

| Medication (oral drugs) | Dosage | Indications/Actions | Contraindications/Notes |
|---|---|---|---|
| **montelukast** *Singulair* | **Asthma, seasonal or perennial allergic rhinitis (taken in PM):** 6 mos-5 yrs: 4 mg 1x/day 6-14 yrs: 5 mg 1x/day ≥ 15 yrs: 10 mg 1x/day **Bronchoconstriction, EIA (prevention):** Take 2 hours prior to exercise 6-14 yrs: 5 mg/dose (chewable tab) ≥ 15 yrs: 10 mg/dose (tablet) | **Seasonal/perennial allergic rhinitis, prophylaxis and chronic treatment of asthma, prevention of exercise-induced bronchospasm** *Leukotriene receptor antagonist blocks inflammatory mediators* | **Adverse:** Headache, dizziness, dyspepsia, fatigue, fever. |
| **zafirlukast** *Accolate* | Take 1 hr before or 2 hrs after eating 5-11 yr: 10 mg 2x/day ≥ 12 yr: 20 mg 2x/day **Tablet:** 10 mg, 20 mg | *Prophylaxis/chronic treatment of asthma* | Same as above May alter liver function Monitor INR if on warfarin |
| **zileuton** *Zyflo* | ≥ 12 yr: 600 mg 4x/day (tabs) 1200 mg 2x/day (extended rel) | *Leukotriene inhibitor: Prevents formation of inflammatory mediators* | Headache, dizziness, dyspepsia, fatigue, elevated LFT's (≥ 3x upper limit norm) |

## Bronchodilators: Beta Agonists SABA

| Medication | Dosage | Indications/Actions | Contraindications/Notes |
|---|---|---|---|
| **albuterol**<br>*AccuNeb*<br>*ProAir RespiClick*<br>*Proventil HFA*<br>*Ventolin*<br>*Vospire ER* | See Below | **Bronchoconstriction, Acute and Maintenance**<br>*Stimulates* β1 *(minor),* β2 *(strong)*<br>**Onset:** 5 min. **Peak:** 30-60 min<br>**Duration:** 3-8 hours | **Adverse:** Slight CV and CNS, hyperglycemia, hypokalemia, tremors |

**ACUTE EXACERBATION (NIH/NAEPP GUIDELINES)**

**NEBULIZER:** 5mg/mL (0.5%); 2.5mg/3mL (0.083%), 1.25mg/3mL (0.042%), 0.63mg/3mL (0.021%).
Child: 0.15 mg/kg (minimum 2.5 mg), every 20 min x 3 doses, then 0.15-0.3 mg/kg (up to 10 mg), every 1-4 hrs as needed **or** 0.5 mg/kg/hr by continuous neb.
Adolescents: 2.5-5 mg every 20 min x 3 doses, then 2.5-10 mg, every 1-4 hrs prn or 10-15 mg/hr by continuous neb.

**MDI:** MDI (HFA and DPI): 90 mcg/puff
Child: 4-8 puffs, every 20 min x 3 doses, then every 1-4 hrs prn.
Adol: 4-8 puffs, every 20 min (up to 4 hrs), then every 1-4 hrs prn.

**SEE ALSO CONTINUOUS NEBULIZER SECTION**

**NON-ACUTE (MAINTENANCE)**

**NEBULIZER:**
Child < 12 yrs: 0.15-0.25mg/kg (max 5mg), every 4-6 hrs prn
> 12 yrs: 2.5-5 mg, every 4-6 hrs prn

**MDI:**
Child < 12 yrs: 1-2 puffs 4x/day
Child > 12 yrs – Adult: 2-4 puffs, every 4-6 hrs (max 12 puffs/day)

**ORAL:**
2-6 yrs: 0.1-0.2 mg/kg/dose, 3x/day (max 12 mg/day)
6-12 yrs: 2 mg/dose, 3-4x/day,
   extended release 4 mg, 2x/day (max 24 mg/day)
> 12 yrs – Adults: 2-4 mg/dose, 3-4x/day, extended release
   4-8 mg, 2x/day (max 32 mg/day)

## Bronchodilators: Beta Agonists SABA

| Medication | Dosage | Indications/Actions | Contraindications/Notes |
|---|---|---|---|
| **levalbuterol**<br><br>Xopenex<br>Xopenex HFA | See Below | **Bronchoconstriction**<br>*R-isomer form of alb-uterol, stimulates Beta-2 (strong)*<br><br>**Onset:** 15 min  **Dur:** 5-8 hrs<br>**Peak:** 1.5 hr | **Adverse:** Slight CV and CNS effects *(less than with albuterol)*, hyperglycemia, hypokalemia<br><br>Risk of paradoxical bronchospasm |
| | **ACUTE EXACERBATION (NAEPP)**<br>**Nebulizer:** 0.31 mg/3 mL, 0.63 mg/3mL, 1.25 mg/3 mL, 1.25/0.5 mL (concentrated dose)<br>Child: 0.075 mg/kg (minimum 1.25 mg) every 20 min x 3 doses, then 0.75-0.15 mg/kg (up to 5 mg) every 1-4 hrs as needed<br>Adult: 1.25-2.5 mg every 20 min x 3 doses, then 1.25-5 mg every 1-4 hours as needed<br><br>**MDI:** (45 mcg/spray)<br>Child: 4-8 puffs every 20 mins x3, then every 1-4 hrs as needed<br>Adult: 4-8 puffs every 20 mins for up to 4 hours, then every 1-4 hrs as needed | **NON-ACUTE (MAINTENANCE)**<br>**Nebulizer:**<br>0-4 yrs: 0.31-1.25 mg every 4-6 hrs as needed<br>≥ 5 yrs: 0.31-0.63 mg every 8 hrs as needed<br><br>**MDI:**<br>≥ 5 yrs: 2 inh every 4-6 hrs as needed | |

| Medication | Dosage | Indications/Actions | Contraindications/Notes |
|---|---|---|---|
| **terbutaline**<br><br>*Brethaire*<br>*Brethine*<br>*Bricanyl* | **Not typically used clinically today**<br>**1 mg/mL**<br><br>**Oral:**<br>< 12 yrs: 0.05 mg/kg 3x/day (max 5 mg/day)<br>12-15 yrs: 2.5 mg 3x/day (max 7.5 mg/day)<br>> 15 yrs: 5 mg 3x/day; reduce to 2.5 mg 3x/day<br><br>**Continuous IV:** 2-10 mcg/kg loading dose, then<br>(asthma)       0.08-0.4 mcg/kg/min<br>            titrate up to 10 mcg/kg/min<br><br>**Continuous Neb** (uncommon):<br>     0.2-0.6 mg/kg/hr | **Bronchoconstriction**<br>**Off Label: preterm labor**<br><br>*Stimulates β-1 (mild),*<br>*β-2 (mod)* | **Adverse:** Slight CV and CNS, hyperglycemia, hypo-kalemia, tremors<br><br>Risk of paradoxical bronchospasm<br><br>More common adverse effects in pediatrics: congestion, cough, fever, rhinorrhea |

7-14

# Bronchodilators: Beta Agonists LABA

| Medication | Dosage | Indications/Actions | Contraindications/Notes |
|---|---|---|---|
| salmeterol<br><br>*Serevent Diskus* | **POWDER:** (50 mcg/dose)<br>≥ 4 yrs: 1 inh 2x/day, 12 hrs apart for:<br>Asthma (>4 yrs; maintenance and prevention)<br><br>**PREVENTION OF EIB (> 4yrs):**<br>1 inh (50 mcg) at least 30 minutes prior to exercise. Don't repeat within 12 hrs, and not to be used by patients on salmeterol 2x/day<br>Chronic use is discouraged (NAEPP) | **Long-Term management of Bronchoconstriction**<br><br>*Long acting selective β2 agonist.*<br><br>**Onset:** 10-20 min<br>**Peak:** 3 hrs.<br>**Duration:** 12 hrs. | **Adverse:** slight CV/CNS<br><br>NOT indicated for acute constriction<br><br>**Black Box Warning**<br>**(see pg 7-9)** |

## Anticholinergics

| Medication | Dosage | Indications/Actions | Contraindications/Notes |
|---|---|---|---|
| ipratropium bromide<br><br>*Atrovent*<br>*Atrovent HFA* | **ACUTE EXACERBATION**<br>**Solution for Nebulization**<br>(0.02%) (0.5 mg/2.5 mL)<br>**Neo:** 25 mcg/kg/dose 3x/day<br>or set: 175 mcg/dose 3x/day<br>**< 12 yr:**<br>  0.25-0.5 mg, 3-4x/day<br>**≥ 12 yr:** 0.25 mg every 6 hrs<br>**Adult:** 0.5 mg every 20 min<br>  x 3 doses, then as needed<br>  (give with SABA)<br><br>**MDI (HFA):** (17 mcg/puff)<br>**Neo:** 4 puffs/dose every 6-8 hrs<br>  (dose given as 4 puffs or 2<br>  puffs, then 2 puffs in 20 min)<br>**< 12 yr:** 1-2 puffs, 3x/day<br>  (max 12/day)<br>**> 12 yr:** 2-3 puffs, 6x/day<br>  (max 12/day) | FDA approved 12+ yrs old<br>Used to treat broncho-<br>spasm in asthma; broncho-<br>dilation in BPD and RDS<br>*Anticholinergic: blocks*<br>*acetylcholine +*<br>*potentiates β2 stim*<br><br><br>**Asthma Maintenance (Non-Acute):**<br>*(GINA, NIH do not recommend)*<br>**Nebulizer**<br>< 12 yr: 0.25-0.5 mg every 6-8 hrs<br>≥ 12 yrs: 0.25 mg every 6 hours<br><br>**MDI (HFA):**<br>< 12 yrs: 1-2 inh every 6 hrs (max 12/day)<br>≥ 12 yrs: 2-3 inh every 6 hrs (max 12/day) | **Adverse:** mucus viscosity,<br>local inflammation, dry<br>mouth, pupil dilation<br>Use mouthpiece when pos-<br>sible to avoid eye contact<br><br>**Not to be used as a<br>rescue inhaler** |

| Medication | Dosage | Indications/Actions | Contraindications/Notes |
|---|---|---|---|
| **tiotropium bromide**<br><br>*Spiriva<br>Respimat* | **MDI (RESPIMAT):** 1.25, 2.5 mcg<br><br>Asthma: 2 inh daily | Maintenance tx of Asthma<br>Action same as Atrovent | **Adverse:** dry mouth, urinary retention, constipation, increased HR, blurred vision, glaucoma<br><br>**Not to be used as a rescue inhaler** |

# Methyxanthines

| Medication | Dosage | Indications/Actions | Contraindications/Notes |
|---|---|---|---|
| **aminophylline** | **NEONATAL APNEA:**<br>Load: 5 mg/kg over 30″<br>(IV or PO)<br>Maintenance: 5 mg/kg/day,<br>q 12 hrs<br>**BRONCHODILATION:**<br>Load: 6 mg/kg over 20-30 min (IV)<br>**Maintenance:**<br><br>**Neonate:** 0.2mg/kg/hr;<br>**6 wk - 6 mo:** 0.5mg/kg/hr<br>**6mo – 12mo:** 0.6-0.7 mg/kg/hr | **Bronchoconstriction**<br>Neonatal apnea<br>**Bronchodilation**<br>(inhibits phospho-<br>diesterase)<br><br>*Stimulates rate and depth<br>of resp., pulm. vasodilation*<br><br>**1-9 yrs:** 1-1.2 mg/kg/hr<br>**9-12 yrs:** 0.9 mg/kg/hr (+ young smokers)<br>**>12 yrs:** 0.7 mg/kg/hr (+ older nonsmokers) | ↑CV and CNS effects, many systemic effects<br>Toxicity > 20 mg/L<br>(> 15 mg/L in neonates) |

## Anti-Infectives

| Medication | Dosage | Indications/Actions | Contraindications/Notes |
|---|---|---|---|
| aztreonam<br><br>*Cayston* | **Powder for Reconstitution:**<br>Oral inhalation (75 mg)<br><br>≥ 7 yrs: 75 mg 3x/day x 28 days (doses should be at least 4 hrs apart)<br><br>*Do not repeat for 28 days after completion. Repeat in cycles of 28 days on, 28 days off.* | Management of *P. aeruginosa* infection in cystic fibrosis | Administer bronchodilator first<br><br>Reconstitute immediately prior to administering (becomes toxic if it sits). Add diluent to powder, gently swirl.<br><br>Administer alone (do not mix with other nebulized meds). Should administer via Altera Neb. |
| colistimethate Na<br><br>*Coly-Mycin* | **Solution for Nebulization:**<br>75mg/mL<br><br>50-150 mg in 3 mL of NS every 8-12 hours. Note TOTAL VOLUME of 4 mL | **Management of P. aeruginosa**<br><br>*Antibiotic for G-activity (pseudomonal activity)* | Reconstitute colistin, diluting dose to 4 mL<br><br>Administer via Pari LC plus nebulizer & filter valve set<br><br>Mix immediately before admin. |

| Medication | Dosage | Indications/Actions | Contraindications/Notes |
|---|---|---|---|
| pentamidine isethionate<br><br>*NebuPent* | - **5+ yrs:** 300 mg (1 vial), once monthly<br>- **< 5 yrs:** 8 mg/kg/dose (up to 300mg)<br>- Deliver via Respirgard II neb at 5-7 L/min at 50 PSI until gone | Prophylaxis of Pneumocystis pneumonia<br><br>*Anti-protozoan* | **Adverse:** Irritation, cough, fatigue, SOB, bronchospasm, metallic taste, systemic effects<br><br>Mix 300 mg (1 vial) w/ 6mL sterile water<br><br>Administer SABA prior to tx |
| **Note:** Caregiver precautions – administer only in an isolated room with separate air circulating system and neg. pressure. Minimize environmental drug exposure. Wear gown, gloves, mask and goggles. | | | |
| ribavirin<br><br>*Virazole* | **AEROSOL VIA SPAG-2:**<br>**Continuous:** (20 mg/mL)[1] reconstitute 6g vial with ≥ 75 mL sterile preservative-free water 20 mg over 12-18 hrs for 3-7 days<br><br>**Intermittent:** (60 mg/mL)[1] reconstitute 6g vial with 100 mL sterile preservative-free water 2,000 mg over 2 hrs, 3x/day, for 3-7 days | Severe (life-threatening) lower respiratory tract infection (RSV, Influenza A, B, Herpes)<br><br>*Antiviral (RSV/influenza A & B)* | Amer. Academy of Pediatrics recommends use only in life-threatening infections<br><br>Minute Ventilation determines actual drug amount delivered<br><br>Do not use in intubated patients (crystallization in circuit occurs)<br><br>See Note under Pentamidine |

[1] Strength (mg/mL) and dose (mg over hrs) is after reconstitution of drug. Continuous administration may be preferred as it limits caregiver exposure to effects of drug.

| Medication | Dosage | Indications/Actions | Contraindications/Notes |
|---|---|---|---|
| tobramycin<br><br>*Bethkis*<br>*Kitabis Pak*<br>*Tobi*<br><br><br><br><br>*Tobi Podhaler* | **NEBULIZER:**<br>BETHKIS: 300 MG IN 4 ML<br>KITABIS, TOBI: 300 MG IN 5 ML<br>≥ 6 yrs: 300 mg, every 12 hr (at least 6 hrs apart), repeat in cycles: 28 days on, 28 days off<br><br>**DPI (Podhaler):** (28 mg/cap)<br>≥ 6 yrs: 112 mg (4 x 28 mg caps), every 12 hrs, repeat in cycles: 28 days on, 28 days off | **Management of P. aeruginosa and other Gram Negative Organism infections (especially in Cystic Fibrosis patients)**<br><br>*Antibiotic for G- activity (Pseudomonal activity)* | **Adverse:** Malaise, headache, Fever, Nausea, Many Respiratory Effects (notable: bronchospasm, cough, dyspnea, hemoptysis, wheezing)<br><br>**Neb:** Administer in Pari LC neb. Suggested order: SABA, then CPT, then other nebs, then tobramycin<br><br>**DPI:** Use podhaler and blister pack. If giving SABA, give it first (15-90 mins before Podhaler). |

| Medication | Dosage | Indications/Actions | Contraindications/Notes |
|---|---|---|---|
| zanamivir<br><br>*Relenza Diskhaler* | **DPI:** 5 mg/inhalation (blister)<br><br>**Influenza Treatment:**<br>≥ 7 yrs: 2 inh (10 mg) 2x/day x 5 days. Doses on days 1+2 should be 2+ hrs apart. Days 3+4+5 should be 12 hrs apart<br><br>**Prophylactic Treatment:**<br>≥ 5 yrs: 2 inh (10 mg) 1x/day x 10 days (start within 36 hrs of onset of symptoms)<br><br>**Prophylactic Commun. Outbreak:**<br>2 inh (10 mg) 1x/day for 28 days (start within 5 days of outbreak) | **Prophylaxis or Treatment of influenza A or B infection**[1]<br><br>*Antiviral (Neuraminidase Inhibitor) which may be used prophylactically and/or as treatment*<br><br>[1]Note that recommendations (indications) for antiviral prophylaxis and treatment are complex - see the Advisory Committee on Immunization Practices (ACIP) for details | **Adverse:**<br>Malaise, dizziness, fever, cough, sinusitis, change in appetite, etc. Anaphylactic reactions have been reported.<br><br>Use in Diskhaler (breath-activated inhaler)<br><br>If giving SABA, give before Diskhaler<br><br>Not recommended for use in patients with airway disease |

# Cystic Fibrosis Transmembrane Conductance Regulator (CFTR) Potentiator

| Medication | Dosage | Indications/Actions | Contraindications/Notes |
|---|---|---|---|
| **ivacaftor**<br><br>*Kalydeco* | 2yrs-6yrs (use granules):<br>< 14 kg: 50 mg every 12 hrs<br>≥ 14 kg: 75 mg every 12 hrs<br><br>≥ 6 years (tablet):<br>150 mg every 12 hrs | Indicated for the treatment of cystic fibrosis (CF) in patients who have a mutation (G551D and others) in the CFTR gene.<br><br>*A cystic fibrosis transmembrane conductance regulator (CFTR) potentiator* | Adverse: URI, headache, stomach ache, rash, diarrhea, and dizziness.<br><br>Administer before or after consuming high-fat food.<br><br>Not effective with two copies of the F508 mutation in the CFTR gene (most common mutation) |
| **lumacaftor/ ivacaftor**<br><br>*Orkambi* | 6-11 yrs:<br>(100 mg/125 mg)<br>2 tablets every 12 hours<br><br>>12 years:<br>(200 mg/125 mg)<br>2 tablets every 12 hours | Indicated for the treatment of cystic fibrosis (CF) in patients age 6 years and older who have a mutation (F508del) in the CFTR gene.<br><br>*A cystic fibrosis transmembrane conductance regulator (CFTR) potentiator* | Adverse: respiratory (chest pain, dyspnea), ↑ BP, hepatic<br><br>Administer with high-fat foods (eggs, avocados, nuts, butter, peanut butter, cheese pizza, whole-milk dairy products, etc.) |

# Mucoactives

| Medication | Dosage | Indications/Actions | Contraindications/Notes |
|---|---|---|---|
| acetylcysteine<br><br>*Mucomyst* | **INHALATION SOLUTION:**<br>10% (100 mg/mL), 10 mL, 30 mL<br>20% (200 mg/mL), 10 mL, 30 mL<br><br>**Nebulized Dosaging (3-4x/day)**<br><br>| Age | 10% | 20% |<br>| --- | --- | --- |<br>| >12 yr: | 10 mL | 5 mL |<br>| Child: | 6-10 mL | 3-5 mL |<br>| Infant: | 2-4 mL | 1-2 mL |<br><br>10% is administered at full-strength<br>20% may be further diluted with NS or Sterile Water<br><br>**Instilled (every 1-4 hrs):**<br>1-2 mL of 20% or 2-4 mL of 10% | **Tenacious mucous**<br><br>*Mucolytic: breaks mucus disulfide bonds. Decreases mucous viscosity.*<br><br>**Peak:** 5-10 min<br>**Duration:** > 1 hr | **Adverse:** Bronchospasm (administer bronchodilator before use), stomatitis, nausea, rhinitis, unpleasant odor/taste. Overmobilization of secretions<br><br>Administer SABA 10-15 mins prior to administration of acetylcysteine<br><br>Administered in oral form for acetaminophen overdosage. Dosaging for this is beyond the scope of this text. |
| dornase alfa<br><br>*Pulmozyme* | **INHALATION SOLUTION:**<br>3 mos- adult: 2.5 mg, 1-2 x/day<br>(1 mg/mL, 2.5 mL amp) | **Tenacious mucus**<br>**(decreases infection)**<br><br>*Selectively cleaves DNA of purulent secretions* | Same as acetylcysteine --<br>Do not mix or dilute with other drugs (may inactivate drug) |

## Inhaled Epinephrine

| Medication | Dosage | Indications/Actions | Contraindications/Notes |
|---|---|---|---|
| **Racemic epinephrine**<br>S2<br>*Asthmanefrin* | INHALATION SOLUTION:<br>22.5 mg/mL<br>1 (0.5 mL) dose = 11.25 mg (2.25%)<br><br>S2:<br>  0.25-0.5 mL (2.25%) diluted in 3 mL NS<br><br>Stridor (2.25%):<br>  < 5 kg:  0.25 mL/dose<br>  > 5 kg:  0.5 mL/dose<br><br>Asthmanefrin: 1-3 inh of 0.5 mL of 2.25% via EZ Breathe atomizer | Bronchoconstriction<br>Tracheobronchial inflammation (post extubation, croup, etc.)<br>Nasal congestion<br><br>Stimulates:<br>  alpha-1 (mild)<br>  beta-1 (medium)<br>  beta-2 (mild)<br>Duration: ½-2 hrs | Milder effects than epinephrine<br><br>Rebound airway edema, cardiac arrhythmias, chest pain, trembling, dizziness, headache<br><br>Use minimum number of doses to get response. Not recommended for routine management of asthma. |

# Inhaled Pulmonary Vasodilators

| Medication | Dosage | Indications/Actions | Contraindications/Notes |
|---|---|---|---|
| iloprost<br><br>*Ventavis* | INHALATION SOLUTION:<br>10 mcg/mL; 20 mcg/mL<br>Initial: 2.5 mcg inhaled,<br>↑ dose to 5 mcg, 6-9 x/day<br>No more than q 2 hr during<br>waking hrs<br>Max/day: 45 mcg | **Treatment of Pulmonary Artery Hypertension (PAH)**, either primary or secondary:<br>congenital heart disease<br>congenital diaphragmatic hernia<br>neonatal pulmonary hypertension<br>cardiopulmonary bypass surgery | **Adverse:**<br>Coughing, headache, nausea, hypotension, bleeding, bronchospasm<br><br>Use I-Neb or Prodose AAD System |
| Treprostinil | Inhaled:<br>3-9 breaths (6 mcg/breath),<br>4x/day | hemodialysis<br>peripheral vascular disease<br>respiratory distress syndrome | **Adverse:**<br>Hypotension, bleeding, cough, headache, nausea, syncope<br><br>Generally well tolerated in infants |
| Epoprostenol<br><br>*Flolan* | Continuous infusion via<br>nebulizer (reconstituted)<br><br>Initial: 1-2 ng/kg/min<br>Titrate by 1 ng/kg/min<br>every 15-30 minutes<br>Max: 100-150 ng/kg/min | Potent Pulmonary Vasodilator. Inhaled form has more targeted effect (less systemic over IV)<br><br>Further studies are needed to determine | **Adverse:**<br>Hypotension, headache, tachycardia, agitation, diszziness |

## Wetting Agents

| Medication | Dosage | Indications/Actions | Contraindications/Notes |
|---|---|---|---|
| **water** sterile, distilled | **Intermittent or continuous nebulization** | **Thick Secretions** *Humidify/thin/liquefy secretions* | Potential mucosal irritation, over-hydration, bronchospasm |
| **Saline:** Hypotonic (0.45% NaCl) | | *Diluent of drugs* | Same as above Less irritating than $H_2O$ |
| **Saline:** Isotonic (0.9%) | | | Bronchospasm |
| **Saline:** Hypertonic | **Aerosol:** intermittent only (2-5 mL) | **Sputum Induction** *Above + osmotic transudate. Used routinely in Cystic Fibrosis patients as a team of therapies for management of secretions* | Bronchospasm, mucosal irritation, edema, ↑ blood $Na^+$ |

## General Considerations with Inhaled Steroids

- Indicated as an anti-inflammatory for maintenance treatment of asthma. NOT indicated for acute symptoms (consider IV steroids for acute exacerbations)
- Adverse effects include oral candidiasis. Pts should be instructed to rinse their mouths, or if too young, consider swabbing mouth after administration.
- Inhaled steroids should be used at the lowest effective dose after Asthma is controlled.
- Dosing guidelines below have been cross-referenced with NIH, GINA, and Manufacturer recommendations

## Inhaled Corticosteroids

| Medication | Dosage | Contraindications/Notes |
|---|---|---|
| **beclomethasone**<br><br>*QVAR* | **HFA (40 mcg/puff, 80 mcg/puff):**<br>5-11 yrs: 40-80 mcg twice daily<br>≥ 12 yrs: 40-320 mcg twice daily<br><br>NIH Asthma Recommendations: | • Not FDA approved for < 5 yrs<br>• Do not shake HFA cannister before use<br>• Prime HFA cannister by spraying 2x<br>• Use cautiously: there is evidence to suggest a reduction in growth for pediatric patients when taking QVAR |

| Dosage Level | 5-11 yrs | ≥ 12 yrs |
|---|---|---|
| Low Dose | 80-160 mcg/day | 80-240 mcg/day |
| Medium Dose | 160-320 mcg/day | 240-480 mcg/day |
| High Dose | > 320 mcg/day | > 480 mcg/day |

| Medication | Dosage | Contraindications/Notes |
|---|---|---|
| **budesonide** (Pulmicort Respules, Pulmicort Flexhaler) | **Pulmicort Respules (nebulized)** (0.25 mg/2 mL, 0.5 mg/2 mL, 1 mg/2 mL)<br><br>Inf: 0.25 mg twice daily or 0.5 once daily<br>Other ages: 0.25-0.5 mg twice daily or 0.5-1 mg once daily<br><br>**Pulmicort Flexhaler** (DPI)<br>(90 mcg, 180 mcg)<br>6-17 yrs: 180-360 mcg twice daily<br>≥ 18 yrs: 180-720 mcg twice daily | There are nuances in dosing with asthma - see manufacturer information for further information.<br><br>**Respules:**<br>Shake gently with circular motion<br>Do not mix with other drugs<br><br>**Flexhaler:**<br>Prime before first use, but at no other time<br>Do not shake; do not use a spacer<br>Do not exhale through mouthpiece |

**NIH Asthma Recommendations:**

| Dosage Level | ≤ 4 yrs | | 5-11 yrs | | ≥ 12 yrs | |
|---|---|---|---|---|---|---|
| | Respules | Respules | Respules | Flexhaler | Flexhaler |
| **Low Dose** | 0.25-1 mg/day | 0.5 mg/day | 180-400 mcg/day | 180-600 mcg/day |
| **Medium Dose** | 0.5-1 mg/day | 1 mg/day | 400-800 mcg/day | >600-1200 mcg/day |
| **High Dose** | > 1 mg/day | 2 mg/day | > 800 mcg/day | > 1200 mcg/day |

| Medication | Dosage | Contraindications/Notes |
|---|---|---|
| **ciclesonide HFA** (Alvesco) | **HFA** (80, 160 mcg)<br>2-4 yrs: 40-160 mcg once daily<br>5-11 yrs: 40-160 mcg once daily<br>≥ 12 yrs: 80-640 mcg MAX daily<br><br>**GINA recommendations:**<br><br>| Low Dose | 80-160 mcg/day |<br>| Medium Dose | 160-320 mcg/day |<br>| High Dose | > 320 mcg/day | | • Prime inhaler 3x initially and with extended non-use<br>• This inhaler does not require shaking<br>• Dose indicator may not work correctly when dropped: instruct pts to then manually track |
| **fluticasone** (Flovent HFA)<br>(Arnuity Ellipta) | **HFA** (44, 110, 220 mcg/puff)<br>4-11 yrs: 88 mcg, 2x/daily<br>≥ 12 yrs: Initial 88 mcg, 2x/daily<br>Max: 440-880 mcg, 2x/daily<br><br>**NIH Asthma Recommendations:** | |

**GINA recommendations:**

| Low Dose | 80-160 mcg/day |
|---|---|
| Medium Dose | 160-320 mcg/day |
| High Dose | > 320 mcg/day |

**NIH Asthma Recommendations:**

| Dosage Level | < 12 yrs | ≥ 12 yrs |
|---|---|---|
| Low Dose | 88-176 mcg/day | 88-264 mcg/day |
| Medium Dose | >176-352 mcg/day | >264-440 mcg/day |
| High Dose | > 352 mcg/day | > 440 mcg/day |

## Combination: Corticosteroid and LABA

| Medication | Dosage | Summary of Action | Contraindications/Notes |
|---|---|---|---|
| budesonide and formoterol<br><br>*Symbicort* | **DPI:** 80/4.5, 160/4.5 (budesonide/formoterol in mcg)<br><br>5-11 yrs: 80/4.5  2 inh, 2x/day<br>≥ 12 yrs not controlled on low-med dose of steroids: 80/4.5,  2 inh 2x/day<br>≥ 12 yrs not controlled on med-high dose of steroids: 160/4.5,  2 inh 2x/day | **Long-term maintenance treatment of asthma who are not easily controlled with corticosteroid and occasional use of a SABA.**<br><br>*Combines action of systemic corticosteroid and LABA* | **SEE BLACK BOX WARNING**<br>**Adverse:** sore nose/throat, headache, stomach irritation, sinusitis, cardiovascular side effects<br><br>SYMBICORT: Instruct patients to shake inhaler for a full 5 seconds prior to using to mix medications. |
| fluticasone and salmeterol<br><br>*Advair* | **DPI:** 100/50, 250/50, 500/50 (fluticasone/salmeterol in mcg)<br>4+ yrs: 100/50,  1 inh 2x/day<br><br>**HFA:** 45/21, 115/21, 230/21<br>≥ 12 yrs: 2 inh, 2x/day | **Long-term maintenance treatment of asthma who are not easily controlled with corticosteroid and occasional use of a SABA.**<br><br>*Combines action of systemic corticosteroid and LABA* | **SEE BLACK BOX WARNING**<br>**Adverse:** same as Symbicort<br><br>All dosing provided assumes no previous inhaled steroid use. Dosages for pts currently on steroids varies - see manufacturer information for starting dosages. |

# Combination: Corticosteroid and LABA

| Medication | Dosage | Summary of Action | Contraindications/Notes |
|---|---|---|---|
| mometasone and formoterol *Dulera* | HFA: 100/5, 200/5 (mometasone/formoterol in mcg) ≥ 12 yrs: 100/5, 2 inh, 2x/day | **Long term maintenance treatment of asthma** *Combines action of systemic corticosteroid and LABA* | **SEE BLACK BOX WARNING** Same as Above Consider higher dose (200/5) if not adequately controlled at 100/5 x 1-2 weeks |

## Surfactants

| Medication | Dosage | Administration | Contraindications/Notes |
|---|---|---|---|
| **beractant**<br><br>*Survanta* | **Sol: 25 mg/mL (4 mL, 8 mL)**<br><br>**Administer endotracheally:**<br>**Prophylactic:** 4 mL/kg as soon as possible. Max: 4 doses may be given in first 48 hrs of life (at least 6 hrs apart)<br><br>**Rescue:** 4 mL/kg as soon as RDS diagnosis made.<br>Max: 4 doses, at least 6 hrs apart | Warm at Room Temperature x 20 minutes (or in hand for 8 mins) Swirl vial, do not shake<br><br>*Administer through a catheter inserted into the ET Tube*<br><br>*Administer the dose in FOUR 1 mL/kg aliquots. Give each portion over 2-3 seconds, preferably in a total of 4 positions (head-down and right, head-down and left, head-up and right, head-up and left)* | **Adverse:** bradycardia, oxygen desaturation, injuries caused by sudden improvement in compliance (air leak, etc.)<br><br>Beractant is a synthetically modified bovine surfactant extract |

## Survanta Dosing Chart[1] (4 aliquots)

| Weight (grams) | Total Dose (mL) | per aliquot (mL) | Weight (grams) | Total Dose (mL) | per aliquot (mL) | Weight (grams) | Total Dose (mL) | per aliquot (mL) |
|---|---|---|---|---|---|---|---|---|
| 600-650 | 2.6 | 0.65 | 1201-1250 | 5.0 | 1.25 | 1801-1850 | 7.4 | 1.85 |
| 651-700 | 2.8 | 0.7 | 1251-1300 | 5.2 | 1.3 | 1851-1900 | 7.6 | 1.9 |
| 701-750 | 3.0 | 0.75 | 1301-1350 | 5.4 | 1.35 | 1901-1950 | 7.8 | 1.95 |
| 751-800 | 3.2 | 0.8 | 1351-1400 | 5.6 | 1.4 | 1951-2000 | 8.0 | 2.0 |
| 801-850 | 3.4 | 0.85 | 1401-1450 | 5.8 | 1.45 | 2001-2050 | 8.2 | 2.05 |
| 851-900 | 3.6 | 0.9 | 1451-1500 | 6.0 | 1.5 | 2051-2100 | 8.4 | 2.1 |
| 901-950 | 3.8 | 0.95 | 1501-1550 | 6.2 | 1.55 | 2101-2150 | 8.6 | 2.15 |
| 951-1000 | 4.0 | 1.0 | 1551-1600 | 6.4 | 1.6 | 2151-2200 | 8.8 | 2.2 |
| 1001-1050 | 4.2 | 1.05 | 1601-1650 | 6.6 | 1.65 | 2201-2250 | 9.0 | 2.25 |
| 1051-1100 | 4.4 | 1.1 | 1651-1700 | 6.8 | 1.7 | 2251-2300 | 9.2 | 2.3 |
| 1101-1150 | 4.6 | 1.15 | 1701-1750 | 7.0 | 1.75 | 2301-2350 | 9.4 | 2.35 |
| 1151-1200 | 4.8 | 1.2 | 1751-1800 | 7.2 | 1.8 | 2351-2400 | 9.6 | 2.4 |

[1] Dosaging based upon manufacturer information

| Medication | Dosage | Administration | Contraindications/Notes |
|---|---|---|---|
| **calfactant**<br><br>*Infasurf* | **Sol: 35 mg/mL (3 mL, 6 mL)**<br><br>**Administer endotracheally:**<br>3 mL/kg every 12 hours.<br>Max: 3 doses in first 96 hrs of life. | Swirl vial, do not shake<br><br>*Administer through a catheter inserted into ET Tube -OR- through a side-port adapter attached to the ET tube*<br><br>*Administer the dose in TWO 1.5 mL/ kg aliquots. Give one aliquot with right-side down, then the other left-side down.* | **Adverse:** Same as above<br>Visible flecks and foaming are normal<br><br>Discard any unused drug once vial has been opened<br><br>Warming is not needed. Avoid repeatedly cooling dose<br><br>Calfactant is a calf lung surfactant extract |

## Infasurf Dosing Chart[1] (2 aliquots)

| Weight (grams) | Total Dose (mL) | per aliquot (mL) | Weight (grams) | Total Dose (mL) | per aliquot (mL) | Weight (grams) | Total Dose (mL) | per aliquot (mL) |
|---|---|---|---|---|---|---|---|---|
| 600-650 | 1.9 | 0.95 | 1201-1250 | 3.7 | 1.85 | 1801-1850 | 5.5 | 2.75 |
| 651-700 | 2.0 | 1.0 | 1251-1300 | 3.8 | 1.9 | 1851-1900 | 5.6 | 2.8 |
| 701-750 | 2.2 | 1.1 | 1301-1350 | 4.0 | 2.0 | 1901-1950 | 5.8 | 2.9 |
| 751-800 | 2.3 | 1.15 | 1351-1400 | 4.1 | 2.05 | 1951-2000 | 5.9 | 2.95 |
| 801-850 | 2.5 | 1.25 | 1401-1450 | 4.3 | 2.15 | 2001-2050 | 6.1 | 3.05 |
| 851-900 | 2.6 | 1.3 | 1451-1500 | 4.4 | 2.2 | 2051-2100 | 6.2 | 3.1 |
| 901-950 | 2.8 | 1.4 | 1501-1550 | 4.6 | 2.3 | 2101-2150 | 6.4 | 3.2 |
| 951-1000 | 2.9 | 1.45 | 1551-1600 | 4.7 | 2.35 | 2151-2200 | 6.5 | 3.25 |
| 1001-1050 | 3.1 | 1.55 | 1601-1650 | 4.9 | 2.45 | 2201-2250 | 6.7 | 3.35 |
| 1051-1100 | 3.2 | 1.6 | 1651-1700 | 5.0 | 2.5 | 2251-2300 | 6.8 | 3.4 |
| 1101-1150 | 3.4 | 1.7 | 1701-1750 | 5.2 | 2.6 | 2301-2350 | 7.0 | 3.5 |
| 1151-1200 | 3.5 | 1.75 | 1751-1800 | 5.3 | 2.65 | 2351-2400 | 7.1 | 3.55 |

[1] Dosaging based upon manufacturer information

# Pharmacology

| Medication | Dosage | Administration | Contraindications/Notes |
|---|---|---|---|
| **poractant alfa**<br><br>*Curosurf* | **Sol: 80 mg/mL (1.5 mL, 3 mL)**<br><br>**Administer endotracheally:**<br>2.5 mL/kg/dose.<br>May repeat at 1.25 mL/kg/dose every 12 hours x 2 more doses<br>Max total dose: 5 mL/kg | Do not shake; invert solution gently<br><br>*Administer through a catheter inserted into the ET Tube*<br><br>*Administer the dose in TWO aliquots. Give one aliquot with right-side down, then the other left-side down.* | **Adverse:** same as above<br><br>Keep refrigerated<br><br>Warming is not needed. If up to room temp,do not re-cool more than once.<br><br>Poractant Alfa is a natural porcine lung surfactant |

## Curosurf Dosing Chart[1] (2 aliquots - Doses Given are TOTAL Doses)

| Weight (grams) | FIRST Dose (mL) | REPEAT Dose (mL) | Weight (grams) | FIRST Dose (mL) | REPEAT Dose (mL) | Weight (grams) | Total Dose (mL) | per aliquot (mL) |
|---|---|---|---|---|---|---|---|---|
| 600-650 | 1.6 | 0.80 | 1201-1250 | 3.1 | 1.55 | 1801-1850 | 4.6 | 2.3 |
| 651-700 | 1.7 | 0.85 | 1251-1300 | 3.2 | 1.6 | 1851-1900 | 4.7 | 2.35 |
| 701-750 | 1.8 | 0.90 | 1301-1350 | 3.3 | 1.65 | 1901-1950 | 4.8 | 2.4 |
| 751-800 | 2.0 | 1.0 | 1351-1400 | 3.5 | 1.75 | 1951-2000 | 5.0 | 2.5 |
| 801-850 | 2.1 | 1.05 | 1401-1450 | 3.6 | 1.8 | | | |
| 851-900 | 2.2 | 1.1 | 1451-1500 | 3.7 | 1.85 | | | |
| 901-950 | 2.3 | 1.15 | 1501-1550 | 3.8 | 1.9 | | | |
| 951-1000 | 2.5 | 1.25 | 1551-1600 | 4.0 | 2.0 | | | |
| 1001-1050 | 2.6 | 1.3 | 1601-1650 | 4.1 | 2.05 | | | |
| 1051-1100 | 2.7 | 1.35 | 1651-1700 | 4.2 | 2.1 | | | |
| 1101-1150 | 2.8 | 1.4 | 1701-1750 | 4.3 | 2.15 | | | |
| 1151-1200 | 3.0 | 1.5 | 1751-1800 | 4.5 | 2.25 | | | |

[1] Dosaging based upon manufacturer information

Pharmacology

## CNS Stimulant

| Medication | Dosage | Summary of Action | Contraindications/Notes |
|---|---|---|---|
| **caffeine citrate**<br><br>*Cafcit* | **Loading dose** (over 30+ mins):<br>20-80 mg/kg<br><br>**Maintenance dose** (over 10+ mins):<br>5-10 mg/kg/day once daily<br>(start 24-hrs after loading dose)<br><br>Consider increasing dose in increments of 5 mg/kg/day (max: 20 mg/kg/day) if insufficient response | Prophylaxis or Treatment of Apnea of Prematurity in Neonates<br><br>*Central Nervous System stimulant* | **Adverse:** tachycardias, arrhythmias, headache, restlessness, ↑ intraocular pressures at higher doses<br><br>Monitor neonates for NEC<br><br>Note that caffeine also has a diuretic effect |

## Analgesia

| Medication | Dosage | Summary of Action | Contraindications/Notes |
|---|---|---|---|
| **Sucrose**<br><br>*Sweet-Ease*<br>*TootSweet* | **Neonatal:**<br>0.1-0.2 mL of 24% solution (on tongue or cheek) 2 mins before procedure<br><br>**Infants:** Up to 10 mL | Short-term analgesia<br><br>*Analgesic - unknown mechanism (? dopamine)* | **Adverse:** Bradycardia (self-limiting), brief apnea possible |

**Pediatric**

**Resuscitation**

**CONTENTS**

This Chapter is a Summary of the *2015 American Heart Association* Guidelines for Basic Life Support (BLS) and Pediatric Advanced Life Support (PALS).

See the Study Table on page 8-8 for the location of PALS sections covered elsewhere in the pocket guide (look for the heart symbol as above).

# Pediatric Basic Life Support with Systematic Assessment

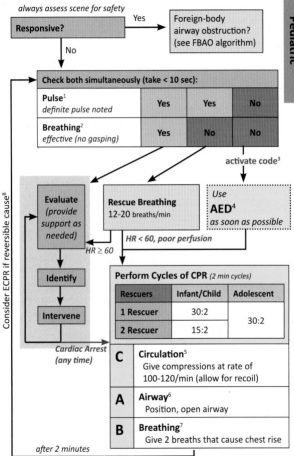

*always assess scene for safety*

**Responsive?** — Yes → Foreign-body airway obstruction? (see FBAO algorithm)

No ↓

**Check both simultaneously (take < 10 sec):**

| **Pulse**[1] *definite pulse noted* | Yes | Yes | No |
| **Breathing**[2] *effective (no gasping)* | Yes | No | No |

**activate code**[3]

Consider ECPR if reversible cause[8]

**Evaluate** *(provide support as needed)*

**Rescue Breathing** 12-20 breaths/min

*Use* **AED**[4] *as soon as possible*

*HR ≥ 60* ↓

**Identify**

↓

**Intervene**

*HR < 60, poor perfusion*

*Cardiac Arrest (any time)*

**Perform Cycles of CPR** *(2 min cycles)*

| **Rescuers** | Infant/Child | Adolescent |
|---|---|---|
| **1 Rescuer** | 30:2 | 30:2 |
| **2 Rescuer** | 15:2 | |

| **C** | **Circulation**[5] Give compressions at rate of 100-120/min (allow for recoil) |
|---|---|
| **A** | **Airway**[6] Position, open airway |
| **B** | **Breathing**[7] Give 2 breaths that cause chest rise |

*after 2 minutes*

**See Further Explanations, Next Page**

## FOOTNOTES
## (see also Summarized CPR Components)

1 **Check Pulse** - "definite pulse OR no definite pulse"
> Take no less than 5, but no more than 10 sec
> Adolescent/child: use carotid or femoral
> Infant < 1 yr: use brachial

2 **Check Breathing** - Simultaneously check breathing with pulse. Note that gasping/agonal breathing is NOT effective breathing.

3 **Witnessed Collapse:** Call code or send someone for help immediately.
> **Unwitnessed Collapse in Peds**: Give 2 mins CPR, then seek help/AED.
>> **Adolescents**: Call code or send someone for help.

4 **AED**: Focus is on use as early as possible but with minimal interruption to chest compressions.

5 **Chest Compressions** — Equal compression/relaxation ratio. Avoid leaning on chest during relaxation phase (may restrict recoil)
> **2 Rescuers:**
>> Unsecured airway - Pause compressions for ventilations. Begin compressions at peak inspiration of 2nd breath.
>> Secured airway - Do not pause or synchronize for ventilations.
>> Change roles every 2 mins to avoid tiring (↓ quality of compressions)

6 **Open Airway**
> *Keep head in neutral position to avoid blockage of airway*
> *Head tilt-chin lift*: preferred when no evidence of head or neck trauma.
> *Jaw thrust:* (primarily for trauma). Open mouth and remove any visible foreign material, vomitus. Blind finger sweeps are NOT indicated.

7 **Provide Ventilation** — Avoid large, rapid or forceful breaths. Do not deliver more volume or force than is needed to produce visible chest rise. Use mouth-to-mouth/nose for infants
> SEE Manual Resuscitation (page 12-6)

8 **ECPR** — Extracorporeal CPR (initiation of extracorporeal circulation and oxygenation during resuscitation). The goal is to support patients in arrest while treating reversible conditions.

## CPR Components, Summarized
### (Infant, Child, Adolescent)

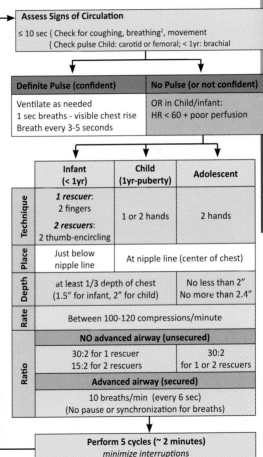

**Pediatric**

**Assess Signs of Circulation**

≤ 10 sec { Check for coughing, breathing², movement
{ Check pulse Child: carotid or femoral; < 1yr: brachial

| Definite Pulse (confident) | No Pulse (or not confident) |
|---|---|
| Ventilate as needed<br>1 sec breaths - visible chest rise<br>Breath every 3-5 seconds | OR in Child/infant:<br>HR < 60 + poor perfusion |

**Resuscitation**

| | Infant<br>(< 1yr) | Child<br>(1yr-puberty) | Adolescent |
|---|---|---|---|
| **Technique** | *1 rescuer*:<br>2 fingers<br>*2 rescuers*:<br>2 thumb-encircling | 1 or 2 hands | 2 hands |
| **Place** | Just below nipple line | At nipple line (center of chest) | |
| **Depth** | at least 1/3 depth of chest<br>(1.5" for infant, 2" for child) | | No less than 2"<br>No more than 2.4" |
| **Rate** | Between 100-120 compressions/minute | | |
| **Ratio** | **NO advanced airway (unsecured)** | | |
| | 30:2 for 1 rescuer<br>15:2 for 2 rescuers | | 30:2<br>for 1 or 2 rescuers |
| | **Advanced airway (secured)** | | |
| | 10 breaths/min (every 6 sec)<br>(No pause or synchronization for breaths) | | |

**Perform 5 cycles (~ 2 minutes)**
*minimize interruptions*

# BLS: Automated External Defibrillator (AED)

| Witnessed Arrest | Unwitnessed Arrest |
|---|---|
| Use AED as soon as device is ready | Initiate CPR<br>Use AED as soon as device is ready |

**Rhythms** (child and adolescent only):
- Shockable Rhythm:
  Give 1 shock, immediately resume CPR (beginning with compressions), do not check pulse. Recheck rhythm in 2 minutes.
- Not Shockable Rhythm:
  Immediately resume CPR. Recheck rhythm in 2 minutes.

**Notes**: Rescuers must practice minimizing the time between compressions to give a shock.

**Infants** (< 1 yr)

| 1st Preference: | Manual Defibrillator |
|---|---|
| 2nd Preference: | AED with pediatric dose attenuator |
| 3rd Preference | AED without a dose attenuator may be used if above two are not available |

**Children**

| 1st Attempt | 2 Joules/kg |
|---|---|
| Subsequent Attempts | at least 4 Joules/kg,<br>*not to exceed 10 Joules/kg*<br>*or the adult maximum dose* |

**Ages 1- 8 yrs**
  use pediatric dose-attenuator system, if available.

# Foreign-Body Airway Obstruction (FBAO)

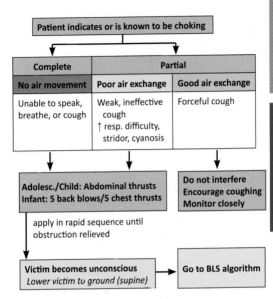

| Patient indicates or is known to be choking | | |
|---|---|---|

| Complete | Partial | |
|---|---|---|
| **No air movement** | **Poor air exchange** | **Good air exchange** |
| Unable to speak, breathe, or cough | Weak, ineffective cough<br>↑ resp. difficulty, stridor, cyanosis | Forceful cough |

| **Adolesc./Child: Abdominal thrusts**<br>**Infant: 5 back blows/5 chest thrusts** | **Do not interfere**<br>**Encourage coughing**<br>**Monitor closely** |
|---|---|

apply in rapid sequence until obstruction relieved

| **Victim becomes unconscious**<br>*Lower victim to ground (supine)* | → | **Go to BLS algorithm** |
|---|---|---|

**Notes:**

*Infant/child –*

5 Back blows/5 Chest thrusts: one every second as needed, same location and technique as chest compressions

Abdominal thrusts not recommended for infants (<1 yr)

*Sudden respiratory distress (coughing, gagging, and/or stridor) accompanied by fever, congestion, hoarseness, drooling or lethargy are indicative of infections such as epiglottitis or croup. The child must be taken immediately to an emergency facility because back blows or chest thrusts will not relieve the obstruction.*

*Late pregnancy (adolescents)* – use chest thrusts

*Obesity* – use chest thrusts (if rescuer cannot encircle abdomen)

# Pediatric Advanced Life Support (PALS) Study Table

# ▦ Pediatric Assessment Triangle (PAT)

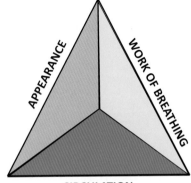

- Rapidly assess 3 areas looking for visual and auditory clues
- Top priority is to determine whether the child is <u>sick</u> or <u>not sick</u>
- A continuous sequence: Evaluate, identify clinical condition, then intervene appropriately. Do not continue assessment if a life-threatening emergency is observed.

**See detailed ABCDE assessment on following pages**

| Assessment Area | Concerning Characteristics | |
|---|---|---|
| Appearance | Abnormal Tone<br>↓ Interactivity<br>↓ Consolability<br>Abnormal Look/Gaze<br>Abnormal Speech/Cry | |
| Work of Breathing | Abnormal Breath Sounds<br>Abnormal Positioning<br>Retractions<br>Flaring<br>Apnea/Gasping | |
| Circulation | Pallor<br>Mottling<br>Cyanosis | Bleeding<br>Purpura<br>Petechiae |

# 5 Categories of Abnormalities (based on PAT)

*Abnormalities in the Pediatric Assessment Triangle suggest an unstable child and require intervention promptly.*

1. Respiratory distress
2. Respiratory failure
3. Shock
4. Central Nervous System/Metabolic disorder
5. Cardiopulmonary failure

## Pediatric Differential Assessment

|  | Appearance | Work of Breathing | Circulation |
|---|---|---|---|
| **Respiratory distress** |  | Abnormal |  |
| **Respiratory failure** | Abnormal | Abnormal | May be abnormal |
| **Shock** | May be abnormal |  | Abnormal |
| **Central Nervous System** | Abnormal |  |  |
| **Cardiopulmonary Failure** | Abnormal | Abnormal | Abnormal |

# ■ ABCDE of Primary Assessment

Pediatric

Resuscitation

**Airway**

- Look for movement of chest, abdomen
- Listen for air movement, breath sounds
- Feel for movement of air at nose, mouth

Goal is to assess for airway patency:

| Clear | Open and unobstructed |
|---|---|
| **Maintainable** | • Signs of obstruction:<br>• ↑ inspiratory efforts (retractions)<br>• Abnormal inspiratory sounds (stridor, snoring)<br>• Apneic episodes with resp. effort |
| **Not Maintainable** | *Differentiate maintainable or not by using basic interventions (see below)* |

**Basic Interventions:**
- Positioning (elevate head)
- Head-tilt/chin-lift if no cervical injury suspected
- Jaw thrust if cervical injury suspected or known
- Suction nose and oropharynx
- Foreign-Body Airway Obstruction (see algorithm)
- Airway adjuncts (e.g. oropharyngeal airway)

**Advanced Interventions:**
- Intubation or placement of an LMA
- CPAP or NPPV
- Removal of foreign body
- Cricothyrotomy

- **Respiratory rate and pattern**
  A sustained RR < 10 or > 60 is a warning sign

| Abnormal Rate | | Possible Causes |
|---|---|---|
| **Tachypnea** | ↑ respiratory effort | First sign of respiratory distress |
| | Baseline respiratory effort<br><br>(Quiet tachypnea) | • High fever<br>• Pain<br>• Anemia<br>• Cyanotic congenital heart disease<br>• Sepsis<br>• Dehydration |
| **Bradypnea** | | • Respiratory muscle fatigue<br>• Central nervous system injury/problem<br>• Severe hypoxia<br>• Severe shock<br>• Hypothermia/hypoglycemia<br>• Drugs that depress respiratory drive<br>• Certain muscle diseases (weakness) |

- **Respiratory effort**
  **Inadequate:** apnea, weak cry/cough, bradypnea
  <u>Nasal flaring</u>: infants, young children
  <u>Retractions</u>:
    Mild-Moderate (subcostal, substernal, intercostal)
    Severe (supraclavicular, suprasternal, sternal)
  <u>Head bobbing</u>: infants in respiratory failure
  <u>Seesaw respirations</u>: upper airway (most often)

- **Chest expansion and air movement**
  **Concerning:** asymmetrical, decreased
  Should be symmetrical and adequate
  Abdomen > Chest may be normal in infants

- **Lung and airway sounds (auscultation)**
  Stridor: upper airway, usually inspiratory
  Snoring: may indicate obstruction
  **Grunting:** sign of severe distress
  Wheezing: lower airway, usually exhalation
  Crackles: fluid vs. atelectasis
  Cry/phonation: cry softens, shorter sentences

- **Oxygen Saturation**
  SpO₂ may indicate hypoxemia early. Both cyanosis and bradycardia are later signs.

  **Interventions**

  | SpO₂ | Indications |
  | --- | --- |
  | < 94% (on RA) | Supplemental O₂ |
  | < 90% (100% O₂) | Supplemental O₂ + Additional Intervention |

  Caution: Abnormal hemoglobins may result in an inaccurate SpO₂. CO poisoning may result in a false high; Methemoglobin results in an SpO₂ ~ 85%

**Circulation**

- **Heart Rate and Rhythm**
  There is a wide range of normal heart rates
  *see page 9-2 for normal rate charts*
  Monitor rate and rhythm (pg 9-9)
  Bradycardia (< 60) with signs of poor perfusion
    requires urgent intervention
  Tachycardia (> 180 infant/toddler, > 160 child)
    with hypotension, mental status change, or signs
    of shock requires urgent intervention

- **Pulses (Peripheral, Central) - see pg 9-8**
  Weak central pulses require urgent intervention

  **The Effect of Shock on Pulses**

  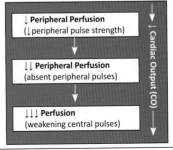

8-13

- **Capillary Refill Time**
  Refill time increases as skin perfusion decreases
  Lift extremity above the heart, press on the skin,
    then rapidly release.  Normal = 2 seconds or less

- **Skin Color and Temperature**
  Normal skin color/temperature should be
    consistent over trunk and extremities
  Changes in hands/feet color/temperature occur
    when perfusion deteriorates
  <u>Pallor</u>: ↓ blood supply to skin, anemia,
    ↓ skin pigmentation
  <u>Central pallor</u>: Anemia, poor perfusion
  <u>Mottling</u>: Vasoconstriction in hypoxemia,
    hypovolemia, shock
  <u>Acrocyanosis</u>: Normal in newly born
  <u>Peripheral cyanosis</u>: shock, CHF, peripheral
    vascular disease, venous stasis conditions
  <u>Central cyanosis</u>: High altitude, alveolar
    hypoventilation, diffusion defects,
    V/Q imbalances, intracardiac shunt

- **Blood Pressure**
  See pg 9-2 for normal blood pressures
    Ensure adequate cuff size (~40% of mid-upper
    arm circumference, extending a minimum of
    50-75% of the length of the upper arm)
  **Hypotension in shock is a sign that normal com-
  pensatory mechanics have failed. Subsequent
  development of bradycardia is an ominous sign
  needing immediate intervention.**
  **Urine Output (mL/kg/hr)**

  | Infants, Young Children     | 1.5 - 2 |
  |-----------------------------|---------|
  | Older Children, Adolescents | 1       |

  Urine output is a sensitive indicator for blood flow
    and perfusion, and is decreased in shock. Note
    that initial measures of urine output may be
    unreliable indicators (there may already be
    urine in the bladder).

- **Neurological Function Assessment**

  **AVPU Pediatric Response Scale**

  | Alert (GCS~15) | Child is awake, active, and appropriately responsive (as age-appropriate) |
  |---|---|
  | Voice (GCS~13) | The child responds only to voice |
  | Painful (GCS~8) | The child responds only to painful stimuli |
  | Unresponsive (GCS~6) | The child does not respond to any stimuli |

  **Glasgow Coma Scale**: See Page 9-12

  **Pupil Response to Light**
  - Pupils should constrict in response to light
  - Pupils should dilate in response to darkness

  **Assess PERRL**: Pupils equal, round, reactive to light

  **Pupils are:**
  - <u>Pinpoint</u>: possible narcotic ingestion
  - <u>Dilated</u>: ↑ ICP, anticholinergics
  - <u>Unilaterally Dilated</u>: Topical absorption of respiratory drug
  - <u>Unilaterally Dilated with Δ Mental Status</u>: Possible temporal lobe herniation

- **Blood Glucose Test:**
  Hypoglycemia leads to brain injury if left untreated.
  *Requires treatment when:*
  ≤ 45 mg/dL newborn
  ≤ 60 mg/dL child

**Exposure**

Undressing the child one area at a time, look for evidence of:

Trauma (bleeding, burns, unusual markings)

Petechiae, purpura, hives

Injuries to extremities (deformities, bruising, tenderness)

## ▬ Secondary Assessment

**Focused History (SAMPLE)**

**S**igns and Symptoms at Onset of Illness

**A**llergies

**M**edications

**P**ast Medical History

**L**ast Meal

**E**vents

**Focused Physical Examination**

Severity of illness/injury should determine extent of exam

**Ongoing Reassessment**

Using Assessment Triangle (see page 8-9) and ABCDE (see pages 8-9, 8-11), review effectiveness of interventions, then return to the triangle

## ■ Pediatric Cardiac Arrest

**Critical Concept:** Most children who go into cardiac arrest do not have underlying cardiac issues. Arrest more often occurs secondary to respiratory failure and/or shock. Clinicians should monitor closely for pending arrest and work quickly to stop progression to full arrest.

### Cardiac Arrest Secondary to Respiratory Failure

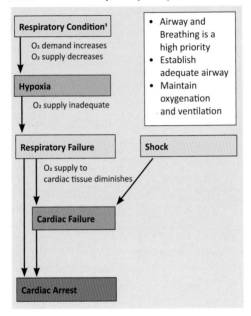

1 Respiratory condition is with or without respiratory distress

## Cardiac Arrest Secondary to to an Arrhythmia

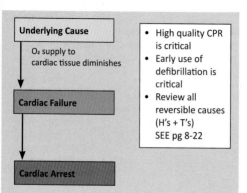

**Underlying Cause**

O₂ supply to
cardiac tissue diminishes

**Cardiac Failure**

**Cardiac Arrest**

- High quality CPR is critical
- Early use of defibrillation is critical
- Review all reversible causes (H's + T's) SEE pg 8-22

# PALS - Cardiac Arrest Algorithm
*(footnotes on following pages)*

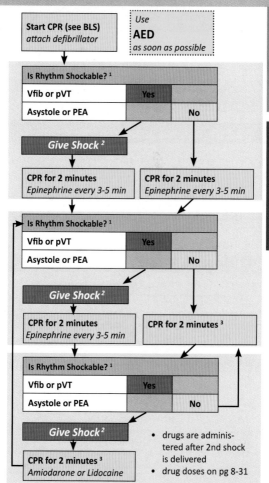

**Start CPR (see BLS)**
*attach defibrillator*

*Use* **AED** *as soon as possible*

**Is Rhythm Shockable?** [1]

| | | |
|---|---|---|
| Vfib or pVT | Yes | |
| Asystole or PEA | | No |

***Give Shock*** [2]

**CPR for 2 minutes**
*Epinephrine every 3-5 min*

**CPR for 2 minutes**
*Epinephrine every 3-5 min*

**Is Rhythm Shockable?** [1]

| | | |
|---|---|---|
| Vfib or pVT | Yes | |
| Asystole or PEA | | No |

***Give Shock*** [2]

**CPR for 2 minutes**
*Epinephrine every 3-5 min*

**CPR for 2 minutes** [3]

**Is Rhythm Shockable?** [1]

| | | |
|---|---|---|
| Vfib or pVT | Yes | |
| Asystole or PEA | | No |

***Give Shock*** [2]

**CPR for 2 minutes** [3]
*Amiodarone or Lidocaine*

- drugs are administered after 2nd shock is delivered
- drug doses on pg 8-31

8-19

**Pediatric**

**Resuscitation**

### Shockable: Ventricular Fibrillation (Vfib)

*Contractions are rapid, unsynchronized, resulting in a muscle that quivers (fibrillates), instead of effectively squeezing.*

### Shockable: Pulseless Ventricular Tachycardia (pVT)

*Abnormal firing of electrical signals, interfering with SA Node. There is insufficient filling time for the ventricles.*

### NOT Shockable: Asystole

*No discernible electrical activity. Often referred to as "flat lined" but is often not perfectly flat.*

### NOT Shockable: Pulseless Electrical Activity (PEA)

rhythm varies but is organized
(p wave, followed by QRS),
or semi-organized

*Organized or semi-organized rhythm with the absence of a pulse. it is an electromechanical dissociation (electrical activity is present, but does not produce the actual pulse).*

## ² Deliver Shock

*Use the largest electrode pads that fit on chest wall without the pads touching. It may be necessary to place one pad on chest wall, one on back (anteroposterior placement), especially with infants.*

| | |
|---|---|
| **Automated External Defibrillator (AED)** | See Page 8-6 BLS: AED |
| **Manual Defibrillator** | Adjustable shock doses<br><br>1. Turn on defibrillator.<br>2. Set Lead switch to paddles<br>3. Select pads or paddles<br>    Paddles: apply gel/paste<br>4. Position:<br>    Pads:  right anterior chest<br>             left axillary position<br>    Paddles: apply firm pressure<br>    Pacemaker:  do not place over<br>5. **Dose:**<br>    **Initial dose:** 2 J/kg<br>    **2nd dose:** 4 J/kg<br>    **Next doses:** 4-10 J/kg<br>     *(do not exceed max adult dose)*<br>6. Charge defibrillator (announce it)<br>7. Clear patient (announce it)<br>8. Shock patient<br>    *Press shock -or-*<br>    *discharge buttons simultaneously* |

- Ensure oxygen is not blowing across infant/child's chest wall during defibrillation
- Always minimize interruptions to CPR. This includes when defibrillator is charging.
- Ensure chest wall is dry (not diaphoretic, etc.)

## ³ Reversible Causes of Cardiac Arrest

| H's | |
|---|---|
| Hypovolemia | Obvious fluid loss? Consider fluid challenge. |
| Hypoxia | Ensure adequate airway (patent?), ventilation (bilateral chest rise?), oxygenation (confirm $O_2$ connected) |
| Hydrogen Ion (acidosis) | Respiratory: Ensure good ventilation<br>Metabolic: Sodium Bicarbonate? |
| Hypoglycemia | Low blood sugar (check level)<br>Treat with IV dextrose |
| Hypo or Hyperkalemia | Hyper: Tall, peaked T-waves,<br>　　　　widened QRS<br>　　　　Give calcium chloride?<br>Hypo: flattened T-waves, prominent<br>　　　U-waves, widened QRS<br>　　　Give potassium |
| Hypo/Hyperthermia | If hyperthermic, cool down<br>If hypothermic, warm up |
| T's | |
| Tension Pneumothorax | Needle decompression needed immediately once identified |
| Tamponade (cardiac) | Pericardiocentesis needed immediately once identified (Chest trauma, central line, JVD, etc.) |
| Toxins | If evidence, find antidote or drug reversal |
| Thrombosis (coronary, pulmonary) | Consider fibrinolysis |

**PALS Special Circumstances:** Drowning, Anaphylaxis, Poisoning, Congenital Heart Disease, Pulmonary Hypertension

# PALS - Bradycardia with Pulse but Poor Perfusion

*if pulseless at any time, go to Cardiac Arrest*

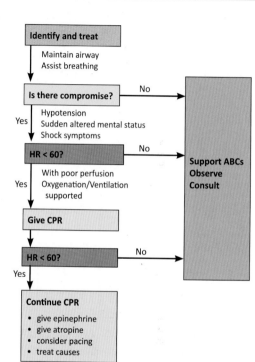

**Identify and treat**

Maintain airway
Assist breathing

**Is there compromise?** — No →

Yes ↓
Hypotension
Sudden altered mental status
Shock symptoms

**HR < 60?** — No →

Yes ↓
With poor perfusion
Oxygenation/Ventilation supported

**Support ABCs
Observe
Consult**

**Give CPR**

**HR < 60?** — No →

Yes ↓

**Continue CPR**
- give epinephrine
- give atropine
- consider pacing
- treat causes

8-23

# PALS - Tachycardia with Pulse and adequate Perfusion

*if pulseless at any time, go to Cardiac Arrest*

**Pediatric**

**Resuscitation**

| Identify and treat | | | |
|---|---|---|---|
| **Normal QRS (< 0.09 sec)** | | **Widened QRS ( > 0.09 sec)** | |
| **Sinus Tach** | **pVT** | **pVT (QRS aberrancy)** | **V tach** |
| Infants: < 220 Child: < 180 | Infants: ≥ 220 Child: ≥ 180 | Infants: ≥ 220 Child: ≥ 180 | Infants: ≥ 220 Child: ≥ 180 |
| P waves present and normal R-R variable PR constant | P waves absent or normal -- -- | -- RR regular QRS unform | -- -- -- |

**Identify and Treat**

**Vagal maneuvers?**

**Vascular access Consider adenosine**

**Expert Consult Identify and Treat 12-Lead ECG Drug Conversion:**
- Amiodarone or
- Procainamide
- Adenosine
(if not given already)

**Electrical Conversion:**
- Consult cardiologist
- Cardioversion
(sedate before)

# PALS - Tachycardia with Pulse and poor Perfusion

*if pulseless at any time, go to Cardiac Arrest*

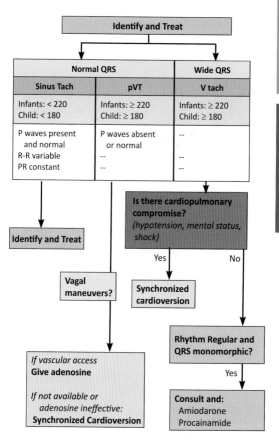

**Identify and Treat**

| Normal QRS | | Wide QRS |
|---|---|---|
| **Sinus Tach** | **pVT** | **V tach** |
| Infants: < 220 Child: < 180 | Infants: ≥ 220 Child: ≥ 180 | Infants: ≥ 220 Child: ≥ 180 |
| P waves present and normal R-R variable PR constant | P waves absent or normal -- -- | -- -- -- |

**Identify and Treat**

**Is there cardiopulmonary compromise?**
*(hypotension, mental status, shock)*

Yes ——— No

**Vagal maneuvers?**

**Synchronized cardioversion**

**Rhythm Regular and QRS monomorphic?**

Yes

**If vascular access Give adenosine**

*If not available or adenosine ineffective:*
**Synchronized Cardioversion**

**Consult and:**
Amiodarone
Procainamide

# ■ Post Cardiac Arrest Care

**Two Phases:**

1. **Immediate**: Focus on immediate life-threatening conditions
   - Airway
   - Breathing
   - Circulation

2. **Management:** Multiorgan care, stabilization, transport

| Airway and Breathing | |
|---|---|
| *Consider NPPV or Invasive Ventilation if unable to meet goals* | |
| **Adequate Ventilation** | • $PaCO_2$ 35-45 mm Hg: titrate as appropriate for the child's condition<br>• Avoid hypercarbia in children with congenital heart disease and pulmonary hypertension<br>• Rapid correction of hypercarbia is unnecessary in respiratory failure and asthma, particularly if on a ventilator |
| **Adequate Oxygenation**<br><br>(↓ risk of reperfusion injury) | • Maintain adequate oxygenation and minimize $FIO_2$<br>  • $SpO_2$ ≥ 94%, but < 100% (avoid hyperoxia)<br>  • $PaO_2$ ≈ 100 mmHg<br>• If not intubated: Use Partial or Nonrebreather until $SpO_2$ confirmed. If $SpO_2$ < 90% on 100% $O_2$, consider noninvasive or invasive measures. |

## student tip

### What is Reperfusion injury?

When there is a period of anoxia or hypoxia, there is an absence of oxygen/nutrients in the blood. This causes damage to cells. This damage is ironically worsened as blood flow is restored (reperfusion). It is thought that this is an inflammatory response. Avoiding hyperoxia may be one way of avoiding some of this additional injury caused by reperfusion.

| Monitoring | • SpO₂<br>• Heart Rate and rhythm<br>• Blood pressure<br>• ETCO₂ (capnography, or colorimetric device intermittently if capnography unavailable) Always confirm ET tube position, then tape and record position at gum/lip<br>• Monitor/assess ET Tube position, cuff pressure if cuffed ET tube. If large air leak around ET Tube, consider larger ET Tube or cuffed ET Tube. PALS recommends keeping most cuff pressures < 20-25 cm $H_2O$. |
|---|---|
| Exam | • Adequate, equal, bilateral chest rise<br>• Abnormal or asymmetric breath sounds<br>• Monitor for respiratory distress |
| ABG | • ABG 10-15 minutes after placing on ventilator<br>• Correlate ABG with ETCO₂ (Record ETCO₂ at <u>time of ABG draw</u> in order to do this) |
| Sedation and Paralytics | • Pain control and sedation should be administered to all intubated patients (who are responsive)<br>• If a child shows poor oxygenation or ventilation, despite adequate pain control and sedation, use DOPE mnemonic to verify no problem (see Student Tip, next page).<br>• If continued difficulty after DOPE, consider NMBA in context of the following indications:<br>  • ↑ PIP/mPAW caused by ↑ RAW or ↓ CL<br>  • Patient-Ventilator asynchrony<br>  • Difficult airway<br>  • **Child should always receive adequate pain control and sedation on NMBA.** Paralytics may mask underlying signs of inadequate oxygenation and ventilation, as well as seizures. |

## student tip

**DOPE mnemonic**
*Sudden Deterioration of Intubated Patient*

| **D**isplacement of tube | Extubated (above vocal cords) |
| --- | --- |
| | Advanced (mainstem bronchi) |
| **O**bstruction of tube | • Secretions, blood, pus |
| | • Foreign body/object |
| | • Kinking of ET tube |
| **P**neumothorax | <u>Simple</u>: sudden ↓ SpO$_2$, ↓ chest expansion and breath sounds on affected side |
| | <u>Tension</u>: Above + hypotension, ↓ CO Tracheal shift away |
| | Other findings may include JVD, pulsus paradoxus, and tachycardia |
| **E**quipment Failure | Multiple possible causes: |
| | • O$_2$ supply disconnected |
| | • Leak in ventilator circuit |
| | • Ventilator failure (power supply, etc.) |
| | • Valve malfunction (bag, vent) |

• Consider manually ventilating patient while assessing DOPE
• Some clinicians add an S to DOPE for asthmatic patients (S stands for *Stacked Breaths*)

| Circulation | |
|---|---|
| *Maintain adequate BP, CO, and distribution of blood flow* | |
| **Monitoring** | • Heart rate and rhythm<br>• Blood pressure and pulse pressure<br>• $SpO_2$<br>• Urine output<br>• Temperature<br>• Consider central line monitoring (ICU)<br>• Consider cardiac function monitoring (ICU) |
| **Exam** | • Repeat physical exam until child is stable<br>• Monitor other systems (renal, neurological) to detect worsening perfusion/circulation |
| **Testing** | • ABG or VBG<br>• Hemoglobin and hematocrit<br>• Glucose, electrolytes, BUN, creatinine, calcium<br>• Lactate, $C\overline{V}O_2$<br>• Chest X-Ray<br>• 12-lead EKG<br>• Echocardiogram (consider) |
| **Intravascular Volume** | • Establish vascular access (2 points of access is preferred)<br>• Fluid boluses as needed:<br>  • 10-20 mL/kg of isotonic crystalloid over 5-20 minutes<br>  • <u>Heart Failure</u>: consider smaller bolus (5-10 mL/kg over 10-20 mins)<br>• **Avoid excess fluid resuscitation** |
| **Blood Pressure** | • **Treat hypotension aggressively**<br>• Maintain post-arrest BP (up to 10 years-old): 70 + ([Age in Years} x 2)<br>• Consider vasopressor (esp. with shock)<br>• Assess hypertension (pain, anxiety, seizures) |

| Tissue Oxygenation | • Ensure adequate oxygenation<br>• Support adequate perfusion<br>• If low hematocrit with signs of inadequate $O_2$ delivery, consider transfusion of packed RBC |
|---|---|
| Metabolic Rate/ Demand | • ↓ WOB: intubate/assist ventilation?<br>• ↓ Pain: analgesia<br>• ↓ agitation: rule out hypoxemia, hypercarbia, poor perfusion, treat with sedation as needed<br>• ↓ fever: antipyretics |
| Arrhythmias | • **Treat aggressively** (tachyarrhythmias, bradyarrhythmias)<br>• Bradycardia: Ensure adequate oxygenation and ventilation. If HR < 60/min with signs of poor perfusion, start CPR<br>• If arrhythmias persist, use drugs or electrical therapy |
| Myocardial Dysfunction | *Common in post-arrest, which may produce hemodynamic instability, organ injury, and ultimately cardiac arrest*<br>• Vasoactives: improve contractility and decrease afterload (BP must be adequate)<br>• Correct abnormalities: acidosis, hypocalcemia, hypoglycemia<br>• Consider PPV (noninvasive or invasive) to improve left ventricular function |

**PALS Drugs**

| Drug | Indications / Mode of Action | Dosing/Administration | Administration Notes |
|------|------------------------------|------------------------|----------------------|
| Adenosine | Supraventricular Tachycardia (SVT) | ***RAPID PUSH:*** IV/IO: 0.1 mg/kg (max initial = 6 mg) <br><br> *If no effect:* IV/IO: 0.2 mg/kg (max initial = 12 mg) | Administer as rapidly as possible |
| Amiodarone | Tachyarrhythmias (various) <br> Ventricular Fibrillation (VF) <br><br> Blocks α and β activity, affecting Na+, K+, and Ca++ channels | Load: 5 mg/kg over 20-60 mins (max 300 mg/dose) <br><br> Repeat doses: 5 mg/kg (max: 15 mg/kg/day) <br><br> *DO NOT GIVE MORE THAN 2.2 g in 24 hours* | |

| Drug | Indications Mode of Action | Dosing/Administration | Administration Notes |
|------|---------------------------|----------------------|---------------------|
| Atropine | Bradycardia (some) Chronotropic (↑ HR) | <u>IV/IO</u>: 0.02 mg/kg (max 0.5 mg/dose) <u>ETT</u>: 0.04-0.06 mg/kg | |
| Epinephrine | Bradycardia VF/pVT Asystole, PEA α = Vasoconstriction β = ↑ HR, Contractility | <u>IV/IO</u>: 0.01 mg/kg (0.1 mL/kg) <u>ETT</u>: 0.1 mg/kg (0.1 mL/kg) *For persistent bradycardia:* IV cont: 0.1-0.3 mcg/kg/min, then titrate to response | Repeat every 3-5 minutes High doses may be harmful |

| Drug | Indications / Mode of Action | Dosing/Administration | Administration Notes |
|------|------------------------------|------------------------|----------------------|
| Procainamide | **Atrial and Ventricular arrhythmias (various)**<br><br>Blocks sodium channels prolonging atrial and ventricular refractory periods.<br><br>Prolongs QT, QRS, and PR intervals | Load: 15 mg/kg over 30-60 mins | Monitor ECG continuously<br>Monitor BP frequently<br>Infuse slowly to avoid toxicity from heart block, hypotension, prolonging of QT interval<br>May increase risk of polymorphic VT |

## Assessment

## Monitoring

# Assessment

## Pediatric Vitals

### Normal Vital Signs Summary Table
*(see following pages for more detailed information)*

| | BP *(mm Hg)* | | HR *(beats/min)* | RR *(breaths/ min)* |
|---|---|---|---|---|
| | Sys/Dia (Mean) | Hypo-tension | | |
| **Infant** *1-12 mos* | 72-104/ 37-56 (45-60) | < 70 | 100-180 (awake) 90-160 (asleep) | 30-53 |
| **Toddler** *1-2 yrs* | 86-106/ 42-63 (49-62) | | 98-140 (awake) 80-120 (asleep) | 22-37 |
| **Preschool** *3-5 yrs* | 89-112/ 46-72 (58-69) | < 70 + (age in years x 2) | 80-120 (awake) 65-100 (asleep) | 20-28 |
| **School-age** *6-9 yrs* | 97-115/ 57-76 (66-72) | | 75-118 (awake) 58-90 (asleep) | 18-25 |
| **Pre-adolescent** *10-12 yrs* | 102-120/ 61-80 (71-79) | < 90 | | |
| **Adolescent** *12+ yrs* | 110-131/ 64-83 (73-84) | < 90 | 60-100 (awake) 50-90 (asleep) | 12-20 |

| **Temperature** | 36.5 - 37.0 C |
|---|---|

## ▣ Respiratory Rate

| | Concerning Bradypnea | RR² (breaths/min) | Concerning Tachypnea |
|---|---|---|---|
| **Infant** 1-12 mos | | 30-53 | |
| **Toddler** 1-2 yrs | | 22-37 | |
| **Preschool** 3-5 yrs | | 20-28 | |
| **School-age** 6-7 yrs | < 10 | | > 60 |
| **Pre-adolescent** 10-12 yrs | | 18-25 | |
| **Adolescent** 12+ yrs | | 12-20 | |

- Assess RR before doing any other hands-on assessment
- A RR < 10 or > 60 in any child is abnormal and requires assessment
- Count chest rise and fall for 30 seconds, multiply x 2
- It can be difficult to accurately count RR using chest excursion in small, tachypneic infants. Use of a stethoscope is recommended, although the touch may increase RR.
- Irregular respiratory patterns (usually containing periods of apnea) are common with neurological problems

## ■ Respiratory Effort

**Pediatric**

### Retractions

| Severity | Retraction | Description |
|----------|-----------|-------------|
| **Mild-to-Moderate** | Subcostal | just below rib cage also called "belly breathing" |
| | Intercostal | between ribs |
| | Substernal | just below the sternum |
| **Severe** *Head bobbing and Seesaw respirations may accompany* | Sternal | sternum towards the spine |
| | Supra-clavicular | above clavicles |
| | Suprasternal | mid-neck, above sternum, also called "tracheal tug" |

**Assessment**

### Respiratory Distress by Retraction and Other Signs

| Type of Problem | Possible Signs |
|-----------------|----------------|
| **Upper airway obstruction** | Retractions *(especially suprasternal, supraclavicular)* Stridor or inspiratory snoring Seesaw respirations |
| **Lower airway obstruction** | Retractions *(especially substernal, subcostal)* Expiratory wheezing |
| **Lung Disease** | Retractions *(especially substernal, subcostal)* Grunting Labored breathing |

## Other Indicators of Respiratory Effort

**Head Bobbing**
More common in infants, involves the use of accessory muscles to
   breathe, a sign of impending respiratory failure

**Seesaw Respirations**
Inspiration: chest retracts, abdomen expands
Expiration: chest expands, abdomen retracts
Note: in neonates and very young infants, some seesaw
   respirations are normal

**Chest Expansion**
Check for symmetry and adequate chest rise (barely noticeable
   through clothing is normal)

**Grunting/Nasal Flaring**
Found in infants primarily, both indicate respiratory distress

**See Also:  Skin Color, Neurological Evaluation**

## Measuring Respiratory Effort and Rate

**Impedance Pneumonography**
An electrical current is passed in between 2 ECG electrodes (placed
   on chest at mid-axillary lines).  This current changes as the chest
   rises and falls, which is then interpreted as a respiratory rate.

<u>Indications</u>:  Monitor respiratory rate, depth, and apnea.

<u>Complications</u>:  May pick up heartbeat and register as a respiratory
   rate (cardiac oscillations); can not distinguish between breathing
   and movement (seizures, obstructive apnea, etc.)

## ▨ Respiratory Distress and Failure

**Goal:** Intervene as early as possible in process to prevent progression to Respiratory Failure

| Respiratory Distress | |
|---|---|
| **Mild** | Tachypnea (mild)<br>↑ Respiratory effort<br>   nasal flaring<br>   retractions (mild) |
| **Severe** | Tachypnea (marked)<br>Tachycardia<br>↑ or ↓ Respiratory effort<br>   retractions (moderate)<br>Poor air movement (distal)<br>Cyanosis<br>Hypoxemia<br>   (even with $O_2$ administration)<br>Agitation |
| **Probable Respiratory Failure** | Abnormal Respiratory Rate<br>   (very rapid, low, or apneic)<br>Tachycardia (severe) - or -<br>Bradycardia (life-threatening)<br>Abnormal respiratory effort<br>   (↑, ↓, or absent)<br>Absent air movement (distal)<br>Cyanosis<br>Hypoxemia<br>   (even with $O_2$ administration)<br>Lethargic |
| **Respiratory Failure** | |
| **Cardiac Failure** | |

## Upper vs Lower Airway Obstruction / Lung Tissue Disease

| | Possible Signs | Causes | Management |
|---|---|---|---|
| **Upper Airway** | ↑ RR<br>↑ Respiratory effort (flaring, retractions)<br>↓ Air movement<br>Breath sounds (↓, stridor)<br>Voice sounds (hoarse, barking cough, snoring, gurgling)<br>Drooling<br>Hypoxemia | Congenital anomaly<br>Foreign body airway obstruction<br>Infection<br>Mass/tumor<br>Secretions<br>Swelling (anaphylaxis, croup, epiglottitis)<br>Trauma (intubation)<br>↓ LOC (tongue, occiput/flexion) | Allow child a position of comfort<br>Minimize agitation<br>Remove foreign body<br>Suction nose/mouth (only if necessary)<br>Drugs (albuterol, epinephrine, steroids)<br>Oxygen<br>Advanced airway?<br>NPPV? Heliox? |
| **Lower or Lung Tissue Disease** | ↑ RR (↓ in severe asthma)<br>↑ respiratory effort (flaring, retractions, ↑, active TE)<br>↓ Air movement<br>Breath sounds (↓, crackles, wheezing)<br>Voice sounds (grunting)<br>Cough<br>Hypoxemia | Pediatric ARDS<br>Asthma<br>Bronchiolitis<br>Congestive heart failure<br>Pneumonia<br>Others (there are many) | See specific disease in disease chapter |

# Cardiovascular
*See Summary Table 9-2 for Rates*

## ■ Central vs Peripheral Pulses

**Central Pulses**                    **Peripheral Pulses**

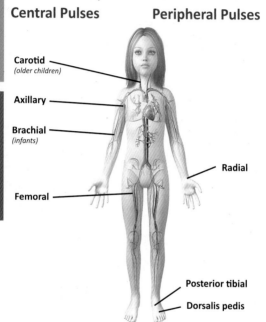

**Carotid**
*(older children)*

**Axillary**

**Brachial**
*(infants)*

**Radial**

**Femoral**

**Posterior tibial**

**Dorsalis pedis**

- Both central and periperhal pulses should be palpated. Heart rate and rhythm should be assessed in context of the child's activity level, clinical condition, and underlying pathologies
- Exaggerated difference between central and peripheral pulses suggests shock (vasoconstriction causes peripheral pulses to become weaker)
- **Weak central pulses require rapid intervention to prevent cardiac arrest**

## ■ Abnormal Pulses and Common Causes

| Type | Possible Cause(s) |
|---|---|
| **Absent** *(in legs)* | Coarctation of the aorta |
| **Weak** | Dehydration <br> Hypovolemia <br> Shock |
| **Weak** *(with slow upstroke)* | Aortic stenosis <br> Coarctation of the aorta <br> Congestive cardiomyopathy |
| **Bounding pulse** *(rapid and strong)* | ↑ ICP <br> Systemic A-V fistula <br> Anemia <br> Aortic insufficiency <br> Hyperthyroidism (Graves' Disease) |
| **Pulsus alternans** *(regular rhythm, alternating strong and weak beats)* | Myocardial failure |
| **Pulsus paradoxus** *(weak on inspiration, strong on exhalation)* <br><br> *MEDICAL EMERGENCY* | Cardiac tamponade <br> Constrictive pericarditis <br> Pericardial effusion <br> Severe Pediatric ARDS <br> Severe air trapping <br> Status Asthmaticus |
| **Dicrotic** *(double pulse; strong/weak)* | Fever <br> Toxemia |
| **Pulsus bigeminus** *(2 beats close together/coupled)* | PVCs |

ICP = Intracranial Pressure
PARDS = Pediatric Acute Respiratory Distress Syndrome
PVC = Premature Ventricular Contraction

# ▇ Blood Pressure Assessment

## Noninvasive Measurement

### *Blood Pressure Cuff (sphygmomanometer)*
Cuff size is critical: the cuff should extend 50-75% of the length of the upper arm
- Cuff too narrow: falsely high measurements
- Cuff too wide: falsely low measurements
- Cuff too tight: inaccurate measurements
- Cuff too loose: falsely high measurements

Measurement should be obtained at the level of the heart

## Signs of poor perfusion in infants and children
- Change in responsiveness
- Skin cool to touch
- Delayed capillary refill
- Diminished pulses
- Evidence of organ failure
- Metabolic acidosis or ↑ serum lactate
- Oliguria (< 1 mL/kg/hr)
- Pale or mottled color
- Tachycardia
- Late signs (impending failure): ↓ BP, ↓ HR

### Estimated Circulating Blood Volume in Children

| Age | Volume (mL/kg) |
|-----|----------------|
| Neonate | 85-90 |
| Infant | 75-80 |
| Child | 70-75 |
| Adolescent | 65-70 |

## Invasive Assessment

(Arterial Line, Central Line, Pulmonary Artery Line)

**Pediatric Differences Affecting Invasive Monitoring**

| Difference | Potential Effect(s) |
|---|---|
| Smaller Vessels | More easily occlude |
| Smaller Measurements | Small errors can result in significant variations from actual |
| Small Blood Volume | There is a critical importance in minimizing blood loss when taking samples, as even a small blood loss can be significant |
| Immunological Immaturity | Increases risk of infection |
| Less Able to Comprehend Procedures | May lead to more anxiety and combativeness. (which may alter measurements) |
| Vigorous Movement of Extremities | Tubes and lines may become dislodged more easily than with most adults (careful positioning and possible restraint is necessary) |

**Detailed information on invasive monitoring, including:**
- Arterial Lines
- Central Lines
- Pulmonary Artery Lines

can be found in
**Oakes' Hemodynamic Monitoring Pocket Guide**
(Dana Oakes, Health Educator Publications, Inc.).

## Neurological Evaluation

**AVPU Pediatric Response Scale**

| **Alert** | (awake, active, responsive) |
|---|---|
| **Voice** | (responds only to voice) |
| **Painful** | (responds only to pain) |
| **Unresponsive** | (doesn't respond to anything) |

**Modified Glasgow Coma Scale**
Scale from 3 (comatose) to 15 (fully alert)

| Adolescent/<br>Older Children | Score | Infant/<br>Young Children |
|---|---|---|
| **Eye Opening** | | |
| Spontaneous | 4 | Spontaneous |
| To speech | 3 | To loud noise |
| To pain | 2 | To pain |
| Not at all | 1 | Not at all |
| **Verbal Response** | | |
| Oriented | 5 | Smiles, coos, cries appropriately |
| Confused | 4 | Irritable and cries |
| Inappropriate | 3 | Inappropriate crying |
| Incomprehensible | 2 | Grunts and moans |
| None | 1 | None |
| **Motor Response** | | |
| Obeys commands | 6 | Spontaneous movement |
| Localizes pain | 5 | Withdraws to touch |
| Withdraws from pain | 4 | Withdraws from pain |
| Flexion to pain | 3 | Flexion to pain |
| Extension to pain | 2 | Extension to pain |
| None | 1 | None |

## Pediatric Early Warning Score (PEWS)

*Score starting with most severe parameters*

|  | 0 | 1 | 2 | 3 |
|---|---|---|---|---|
| **Behavior** | Appropriate to age | Drowsy/ Sleeping | Irritable | Lethargic or ↓ Pain Response |
| **Cardio-vascular** | Pink | Pale or dusky toned | Gray or cyanotic | Gray or cyanotic + mottling |
|  | Capillary refill 1-2 seconds | Capillary refill 3 seconds | Capillary refill 4 seconds | Capillary refill 5+ seconds |
|  |  |  | HR 20 bpm > normal rate | HR 30+ bpm > normal rate (or bradycardia which is a serious sign) |
| **Respiratory** | Normal | RR > 10 above normal | RR > 20 above normal + retractions | 5+ BELOW normal + retractions or grunting |
|  |  | Accessory muscles |  |  |
|  |  | O₂ 30% or 3+ L/min | O₂ 40% or 6+ L/min | O₂ 50% or 8+ L/min |
|  | For HFNC: Use O₂%, not flow in scoring<br>For NC: Use L/min in scoring | | | |
| **Add 2 Points** | IF pt receiving continuous (or frequent) nebulizer treatments OR has persistent postoperative vomiting | | | |

Adapted from Monaghan. Detecting and managing deterioration in children. Pediatric Nursing. 2005 (17)32-35.

# ■ Other

**Skin Color**

| Pallor (Pale) | | Lack of normal color<br>  (skin or mucous membrane)<br>Lips, inside mouth, tongue, eye linings, hand<br>  palms, soles of feet may be clinically significant<br><br>Central pallor:<br>• anemia<br>• poor perfusion<br>General pallor:<br>• ↓ blood supply to skin (cold, stress, shock)<br>• Anemia<br>• ↓ skin pigmentation (can mislead) |
|---|---|---|
| Mottling | | Irregular/pathy discoloration of skin<br>(irregular supply of blood to skin)<br>• Shock<br>• Hypoxemia<br>• Hypovolemia |
| Cyanosis | Acro-cyanosis[1] | Hands/Feet/Mouth are bluish<br>Common in newborns and is characterized by<br>peripheral cyanosis |
| | Peripheral cyanosis[1] | Hands/Feet are bluish (beyond newborn)<br>(diminished oxygen delivery to tissues)<br>• Shock<br>• Congestive heart failure<br>• Periperhal vascular disease<br>• Hypoxemia<br>• Poor perfusion |
| | Central cyanosis | Lips/Mucous Membranes are bluish<br>• Pneumonia or other diffusion defect<br>• Alveolar hypoventilation (TBI, etc.)<br>• V/Q imbalance (PARDS, Asthma, etc.) |

1 Acrocyanosis and peripheral cyanosis are virtually the same thing. Cyanosis is a
bluish discoloration of peripheral areas (caused by reduced hemoglobin in capillary beds > 3 g/dL). Acrocyanosis is considered normal in newborns. Peripheral
cyanosis beyond the newborn period is abnormal and the term acrocyanosis no
longer applies.

**Capillary Refill**

*> 2 seconds is considered abnormal*
- Typical with dehydration, shock, hypothermia

**Skin Temperature**

Use back of hand to check skin temperature - slide up extremity to find spot where it transitions from cool to warm.

This transition line should move towards the hands/feet as the child improves.

## ▨ Other Assessments

**Urine Output**

| Infants/Young children | 1.5 - 2 mL/kg/hr |
|---|---|
| Older children/Adolescents | 1 mL/kg/hr |

- Catheter is most accurate way to measure urine amounts
- Urine output may be an indication of perfusion
- Improved output suggests a response to therapy
- Observe urine color (blood-tinged, bloody, etc.)

# Monitoring 〜♥〜

## ■ Oxygen Monitoring

| Method | Normal Values | Description |
|--------|---------------|-------------|
| **Noninvasive** | | |
| $SpO_2$ | > 95% | Peripheral $O_2$ saturation (measured Hb saturation via Pulse Oximeter) |
| TCM | ~80-100 mm Hg | Transcutaneous Monitoring estimates $PaO_2$ by inducing hyperperfusion (via heating) of skin site and measuring electrochemically |
| **Invasive** | | |
| $PaO_2$ | 80-100 mm Hg | Partial Pressure of Oxygen molecules within blood (not those bound to hemoglobin) |
| $SaO_2$ | > 95% | Calculated $O_2$ saturation from $PaO_2$ (if an analysis), or actual measured value (co-oximeter) |

**Notes:**
- Trends are more important than absolute values
- $SpO_2$ may be a poor indicator of $SaO_2$
- Periodic baseline correlations should be made with $PaO_2$ and/or $SaO_2$ (CO-oximetry)
- Pulse oximetry alone can not indicate hyperoxemia (maximum is 100%)
- $SpO_2$ values may vary between various models of oximeters, so caution in interchanging oximeters on same patient
- Factors affecting $SpO_2$ – See also Next Page

# Pulse Oximetry[1, 2]

### Indications
Need to monitor $SaO_2$,
Need to quantitate patient's
response to therapy or diagnostic procedure.

### Contraindications
Ongoing need to measure
pH, $PaCO_2$, total Hgb, and/or
abnormal Hgb (relative).

### Hazards/Complications
Inappropriate therapy due
to false negative or positive
results, probe misuse (pressure sores, burns, electrical
shock).

### Frequency
Variable depending on clinical status, indications, and
procedures being performed.

### Monitoring
**Validity of reading** –
Compare $SpO_2$ with $SaO_2$
and HR with pulse rate
(initial and periodic).
Document conditions: patient
position, activity level,
site perfusion, probe
location, type of oxygen
therapy.
Check for invalidating factors:
abnormal Hgb, exposure
to light, hyperoxemia, intra
vascular dyes, low perfusion
state, motion artifact, nail
polish/covering, saturation <
83%, skin pigmentation.

**Patient** – vital signs

### Clinical Goal
(desired outcome)
To reflect the patient's clinical, oxygenation condition.

[1] Pulse oximetry ($SpO_2$) is a noninvasive determination of
oxyhemoglobin saturation ($SaO_2$).
[2] Adapted from the AARC Clinical Practice Guideline: Pulse Oximetry,
*Respiratory Care*, Vol. 36, #12, 1991

> Pulse oximetry is helpful in identifying changes in lung function and establishing the need for a change in or discontinuation of $O_2$ therapy.
>
> The Respiratory Care Practitioner must be acutely aware of the potential inaccuracies of oximetry readings and take them into account when recommending changes. Never use oximetry results as the only parameter when making respiratory care decisions.

## Troubleshooting the Pulse Oximeter

| Problem | Possible Cause(s) | Interventions |
|---------|-------------------|---------------|
| **Inaccurate SpO₂** (does not correlate with SaO₂ from ABG) <br><br> *New pulse oximeters are less likely to cause these problems | **Patient** <br> • Movement* <br> • Poor perfusion (cool skin, PVD, etc.)* <br> • Skin pigment (darker)* <br> • High carboxyhemoglobin or methemoglobin <br> • Reduced arterial blood flow | • Encourage pt to be still, if possible or able <br> • Check sensor site - consider moving from one finger to another, earlobe, toe, forehead, nare <br> • Consider replacing sensor <br> • Use other forms of measure if needed to confirm (ABG, TCM, etc.) <br> • Warm site with approved warming device |
| | **Environment** <br> • Cool Room* <br> • Ambient Light* | • Warm site with approved warming device <br> • Cover sensor to block ambient light <br> • Ensure sensor is not distal to BP cuff |
| | **Equipment** <br> • Blood Pressure cuff placement <br> • Sensor not adhering well | • Ensure sensor is placed securely; replace if necessary. <br> • Check sensor site - consider moving from one finger to another, earlobe, toe, forehead, nare <br> • Consider different type of sensor (neonatal, etc.) <br> • Use ECG signal synchronization. <br> • Select a longer (10-15 sec) averaging time, if possible. |

| Problem | Possible Cause(s) | Interventions |
|---|---|---|
| **Loss of Pulse Signal, Poor Waveform**<br><br>*New pulse oximeters are less likely to cause these problems | **Patient**<br>• Reduced arterial blood flow<br>• Anemia<br>• Hypothermia<br>• Shock (hypotension, vasocon)<br>• Nail polish* | • Confirm or follow with ABG<br>• Check Hemoglobin level<br>• Consider warming site, replace sensor<br>• Always check pt's condition, vitals<br>• More likely to intefere if contains metallic flakes, remove |
| | **Environment**<br>• Excessive ambient light* | • Cover sensor to block ambient light |
| | **Equipment**<br>• Constriction by sensor<br>• Sensor is not on patient | • Check sensor<br>• Move to a different site or change type of sensor used<br>• Confirm sensor is on patient |
| **Inaccurate Pulse Rate** | **Patient**<br>• Excessive patient motion | • Encourage patient to be still if able |
| | **Equipment**<br>• Pronounced dicrotic notch on art. waveform<br>• Poor quality ECG signal<br>• Electrocautery interference | • Move sensor to a different site<br>• Check ECG leads; replace if necessary.<br>• Same as above. |

## ▣ Transcutaneous Monitoring

Oxygen (PtcO$_2$) and Carbon Dioxide (PtcCO$_2$) can both be monitored.

### Indications:

- Diagnosis, clinical management, and early idenitfication of cardiac and respiratory problems
- Prevention of hyperoxia/hypoxia, hypercapnia/hypocapnia
- Evaluate response to therapeutic interventions, including non-invasive and invasive therapies
- Monitor effects of apnea, right-to-left shunts, crying, and breath-holding (PtcO$_2$)

### Technique:

A heated electrode (*Clark* for Oxygen, *Severinghaus* for Carbon Dioxide) is placed on the skin surface (the heat arterializes the site and increases permeability to gas diffusion)

### Preferred Sites *(Avoid bony areas and extremities)*:

- Anterior chest
- Abdomen
- Back
- Inner thigh

### Hazards:

- Burns (rotate site every 2-6 hours)
- Values are dependent on barometric pressure
- May underestimate PaO$_2$ in children with chronic conditions (BPD)

### Interpretation

| PtcO$_2$ | reads lower than actual PaO$_2$ (dependent on dissociation curve) |
|---|---|
| PtcCO$_2$ | reads higher than actual PaCO$_2$ (by 2-20 mm Hg) |

- Transcutaneous measures must be correlated with appropriate blood gas values. Draw an ABG, being sure to record transcutaneous values <u>at the time of the blood draw</u>, then correlate.
- Note that PtcO$_2$ is a crude but accurate estimate of PaO$_2$. PtcCO$_2$ is less reliable

# ▨ End Tidal Carbon Dioxide Monitoring

Measure of end-tidal $CO_2$ (ETCO2, PETCO$_2$) which is used as an estimate of $PaCO_2$.

**Indications:**

- Diagnosis, clinical management, and early idenitfication of cardiac and respiratory problems
- Prevention of hypercapnia/hypocapnia
- Evaluate response to therapeutic interventions, including noninvasive and invasive therapies
- Evaluate effectiveness of compressions during CPR (goal is to increase ETCO$_2$ by > 10-15 mm Hg)
- Waveform capnography is helpful in determining severe obstruction (asthma, for example) and the resulting response to therapies

**Technique:**

A collection device is placed either in-line with an invasive circuit (directly in-line, or sampling from in-line) or a catheter near the nares (often in combination with an oxygen cannula)

**Interpretation**

- Under normal conditions ETCO$_2$ closely approximates $PaCO_2$
- Trends are much more important than a single measured value
- Changes in correlation between ETCO$_2$ and $PaCO_2$ can indicate changes in underlying respiratory physiology. ETCO$_2$ may be inaccurate when:
  - Severe respiratory disease
  - Pulmonary emboli
  - Increased deadspace ventilation
  - Increased alveolar ventilation

## ■ Invasive Blood Gas Monitoring

**Venous Blood Gas (VBG) Monitoring**
- Drawing venous blood can often be done from existing catheterization but provides limited information (see table below)
- Assess perfusion of the site (temperature, color, etc.) as drawing to ensure adequately correlated results

**Capillary Blood Gas (CBG) Monitoring:**
- Usually preferred for neonates and small infants. Clinical value is highly dependent on arterialization — careful heating of the site without milking which can lyse cells and alter results
- pH and PcCO₂ correlate well when arterialized, but oxygenation does not correlate reliably

**Correlation of VBG and CBG to ABG Values**

*These are general guidelines. Correlations are subject to individual disease states, perfusion, sample quality, etc. An ABG should be drawn whenever possible in critical care sitatuations.*

| Value | ABG | VBG | CBG |
|---|---|---|---|
| pH | 7.35-7.45 (7.40) | correlates with ABG | correlates with ABG |
| PaCO₂ (mm Hg) | 35-45 (40) | within 4-6 mm Hg | correlates with ABG |
| PaO₂ (mm Hg) | 75-100 | does not correlate reliably | does not correlate reliably |
| SaO₂ (%) | 94-100% | | |
| HCO₃ (mEq/L) | 22-26 | correlates with ABG | correlates with ABG |

# ■ Chest X-Ray Interpretation

## Systematic Approach to Interpreting a Peds CXR

1. **Confirm patient.**
2. **Confirm date and time.**
3. **Identify type:** AP or PA (special: lateral decubitis)
4. **Check quality:** about 4 vertebrae visible, Inspiratory Film?
   Exp film may show abnorm ↑ heart size, ↓ volume, ↑ interstitium
5. **Check rotation:** Anterior rib ends/clavicles centered around vertebrae
6. **Systematically explore from Outside-to-Inside:**

| Soft Tissue | Amount of tissue (obesity, breasts) |
|---|---|
| | Subcutaneous emphysema (crepitus) |
| **Bones** | Examine for fractures, especially clavicles, ribs. |
| | Obvious spinal deformity (scoliosis, etc.)? |
| **Heart** | Size varies by age - generally > 60% is abnormal |
| | Identify: Major structures (ventricles, etc.) |
| **Lungs** | Expansion (7-9 ribs, mid-clavic. at diaphragm) |
| | Find trachea, carina (midline?) |
| | Find fissures, if visible |
| | Find hila (L is above R) |
| | Costophrenic and Cardiophrenic Angles |
| | (blunted ~fluid?) |
| | Diaphragm: Right is slightly ↑ than Left (liver) |
| | Elevated? Flattened (air trap)? |
| | Parenchyma: |
| | Haziness (~atelctasis) |
| | Consolidation (air bronchograms at periphery) |
| | Infiltrates (consolidation, localized or diffuse) |
| | Pneumothorax (lack of vasc. markings) |
| | General abnormalities (foreign objects, |
| | nodules, etc.) |
| **Tubes Lines** | ET Tube |
| | Trach Tube (present or not) |
| | Gastric tube |
| | Chest tube(s) |
| | EKG leads |
| | Central Line / Pulmonary Artery Line |

Pediatric

Assessment

Pediatric

Diseases

CONTENTS

**Pediatric**

**Diseases**

| NAME - MOST COMMONLY ACCEPTED MEDICAL TERM LISTED IN ALPHABETICAL ORDER (OTHER NAMES OR ABBREVIATIONS) | |
|---|---|
| Def | Definition |
| Types | When present, contains information regarding **various types** of disease or disorder |
| Etiology | **Origin** of disease or disease-causing organisms. |
| CM | **Clinical Manifestations** Listings indicate the most commonly found pulmonary manifestations (not all-inclusive). Manifestations of other body systems are generally not included. |
| CXR | **Chest X-Ray** - common findings |
| EBG | **Evidence-Based Guidelines** if available for Topic |
| CC | **Critical Care Considerations** - note that this will indicate material available in other Oakes' Pocket Guides. |
| Tx | **Treatment Overview**, including relevant algorithms based on latest Evidence-Based Medicine |

**Not every category will be presented for every disease - only those that have been deemed clinically relevant.**

| ASTHMA | | | |
|---|---|---|---|
| **Def** | A heterogeneous disease usually characterized by chronic airway inflammation that is at least partially reversible. It is defined by the history of respiratory symptoms (wheeze, SOB, chest tightness, cough, etc.) that may vary over time and in intensity, together with variable expiratory airflow limitation. | | |
| **Types** | **Extrinsic** (allergic) asthma: 90% of all asthma; typically develops in childhood | | |
| | **Intrinsic** (non-allergic) asthma: 10% of all asthma; develops after age of 30 to 40 | | |

| Etiology | | |
|---|---|---|
| **Inhalation** | • Genetic?<br>• **Allergens:**<br>  • Animal (dander, urine, etc)<br>  • Pests (cockroach feces, dust mites)<br>  • Indoor fungi or outdoor pollen, spores<br>• **Environmental exposures:**<br>  • Dust, gases, fumes, chemicals<br>• **Irritants:**<br>  • Air pollution, odors, sprays, stove fumes, tobacco smoke | |
| **Other Factors** | • Cold air, exercise<br>• Emotional stress<br>• Gastroesophageal reflux, food<br>• Rhinitis/sinusitis<br>• Sensitivity to drugs (aspirin, beta-blockers, nonsteroidal anti-inflammatory, sulfites)<br>• Viral respiratory infections | |

| CM | | | |
|---|---|---|---|
| Agitation/restless<br>Anxiety<br>Chest tightness<br>Cough<br>Diaphoresis<br>Dyspnea/SOB<br>Flaring | ↑RR, ↑HR<br>↑TE, ↑WOB<br>Hyperinflation<br>Hyperresonance<br>Hypoxemia<br>Pulsus paradoxus<br>Retractions | Wheezing*<br><br>Late signs:<br>↓$PaCO_2$ (initial)* →<br>  ↑$PaCO_2$ (late)<br>↓ BS<br>Cyanosis | |
| **DANGER:** Respiratory distress without wheezing (silent chest), or ABG with normal $PaCO_2$ (child tiring) may indicate impending respiratory failure | | | |

| | **Is it Asthma?** * |
|---|---|
| CM (cont.) | *The presence of any of these signs and symptoms should increase the suspicion of asthma:*<br>• Wheezing (but don't exclude consideration if not present)<br>• History of:<br>  - Cough, worse at night<br>  - Recurrent wheeze, difficult breathing, or chest tightness<br>• Symptoms occur or worsen at night, awakening patient<br>• Patient also has eczema, hayfever, or family hx of asthma<br>• Symptoms occur or worsen in the presence of<br>  (see etiology above for list)<br>• Symptoms respond to anti-asthma therapy<br>• Patient's colds "go to the chest" or take more than 10 days to clear<br><br>* *Adapted from Global Initiative for Asthma (GINA), 2016*<br><br>**PFTs: Obstructive Pattern**<br>↓FVC, ↓FEV & FEV₁%, ↓PEF  ----  ↑FRC, ↑RV, ↑TLC |
| CXR | Hyperinflation, ↑bronchial markings, flat diaphragm, ↑rib spaces, more radiolucent, narrow heart shadow. |

Arterial blood gas, ABG, during various stages of asthma.

10-4

**EBG**
- *Global Strategy for Asthma Management and Prevention* - Global Initiative for Asthma (GINA), 2016 Includes a quick reference guide and at-a-glance summaries. SEE GINA website (ginasthma.org).
- *International ERS/ATS Guidelines on Definition, Evaluation, and Treatment of Severe Asthma*, 2014

**CC**

See Oakes' Ventilator Management for detailed Mechanical Ventilation strategies related to Asthma

**ASTHMA Tx**

### Levels of Asthma Control*

| Characteristic | Controlled (all of the following) | Partly controlled (any measure present in any week) | Uncontrolled |
|---|---|---|---|
| Daytime symptoms | None (≤ 2/week) | > 2/week | 3+ features of partly controlled asthma present in any week |
| Limitations of Activities | None | Any | |
| Nocturnal symptoms/ awakening | None | Any | |
| Need for reliever/rescue treatment | None (≤ 2/week) | > 2/week | |
| Lung Function (PEF or FEV₁) | Normal | < 80% pred or personal best | |
| Exacerbations | None | ≥ 1 /year | 1 in any week |

*\* Adapted from Global Initiative for Asthma (GINA)*

**Asthma Severity, Control, and Treatment**

**Classifying Severity of Asthma Exacerbations ***

ASTHMA Tx

| Parameter[1] | Mild | Moderate | Severe | Respiratory Arrest Imminent |
|---|---|---|---|---|
| Breathless | Walking, can lie down | Talking, prefers sitting | At rest, hunched forward | |
| Talks in | Sentences | Phrases | Words | |
| Alertness | May be agitated | Usually agitated | Usually agitated | Drowsy or confused |
| RR[2] | ↑ | ↑ | Often > 30/min | |
| Accessory Muscle Use | None | Usually | Usually | Paradoxical Breathing |
| Wheeze | Moderate, end-expir | Loud | Usually loud | Absent |
| Pulse[3] | <100 | 100-120 | > 120 | < 60 |
| Pulsus paradoxus | Absent, < 10mmHg | May be present, 10-25 mmHg | Often present, > 25 mmHg[4] | Absent? = respiratory fatigue? |
| PEF[5] | > 80% | 60-80% | < 60% [6] | |
| PaO2 (on RA) (mm Hg) | Normal | > 60 | < 60 | |
| PaCO2 [7] (mm Hg) | < 45mmHg | < 45 | > 45 | |
| SaO2 (on RA) | > 95% | 91-95% | < 90% | |

1. The presence of several parameters, but not necessarily all, indicates the general classification of the attack
2. Normal RR for children: < 2 mo, < 60/min; 2-12 mo, < 50/min; 1-5 yrs, < 40/min; 6-8 yrs, < 30/min
3. Normal pulse for children: infants (2-12 mo), < 160/min; preschool (1-2 yrs), < 120/min; school age (2-8 yrs), < 110/min
4. 20-40 mm Hg in children
5. After initial bronchodilator, % pred or % personal best
6. < 100 L/min adults or response lasts < 2 hrs
7. Hypercapnia develops more readily in young children than in adults and adolescents

**Treatment Strategies**
**See Severity Chart for details on Symptoms of Distress**

| ASTHMA Tx (continued) | General Therapy<br><br>(Mild to Moderate Symptoms) | • Oxygen Therapy should be given to all pts in respiratory distress<br>• Follow oxygenation via $SpO_2$ or A-Line<br>• Maintain $SpO_2$ > 90%<br>• Aggressive hydration may be indicated for infants/small children, but is not recommend for older children<br>• CPT, mucolytics, routine CXR, ABG, and sedation are not typically recommended<br>• Inhaled SABA and oral corticosteroids |
|---|---|---|
| | (Moderate to Severe Symptoms) | • Continuous SABA, ipratropium bromide, and high dose oral or IV steroids<br>• Consider IV Mag sulfate and/or Heliox for pts not responding to initial tx. |
| | Respiratory Failure | • Do not delay Intubation once indicated<br>• Use of NPPV is controversial, but may support pt's ventilatory needs for a short trial. Do not sedate or use in agitated patients<br>• During BVM, be aware of high risk of air-trapping<br>• May continue Steroids and high-dose bronchodilators when on PPV<br>• Aim for early extubation post-crisis |
| | Post-Crisis | • Utilize opportunity to do comprehensive education post-crisis. Discussion should include use of an asthma plan, patient demonstration of proper use of medications, as well as indications, etc.<br>• Include family supports as appropriate<br>• Include environmental review (triggers)<br>• Connect patient with Asthma Educator/ Program when available. Use bilingual services when available/needed.<br>• Strongly emphasize the controllable nature of Asthma |

## BRONCHIOLITIS
### (INCLUDING RESPIRATORY SYNCTIAL VIRUS [RSV])

| | |
|---|---|
| **Def** | Acute lower airway respiratory infection in the infant, causing inflammation, edema, ↑ mucus production, and bronchoconstriction of the small airways |
| **Etiology** | RSV is a viral infection - the majority of infants develop RSV before the age of 2-years-old (peak = 6 months).  There is an RSV "season" that can occur during fall, winter, or spring in the U.S. - this varies by region. |
| **CM** | **Diagnosis** by history, swab <br>    (nasal wash, nasopharyngeal, throat) <br><br> • Apnea (reflex) <br> • Respiratory distress (retractions, tachypnea, cyanosis, nasal flaring) <br> • Wheezing <br> • Cough <br> • Rhinorrhea <br> • Sinus and Ear involvement are common |
| **CXR** | • Hyperinflation <br> • ↑ perihilar markings or peribronchial thickening (indicates possible bronchial inflammation) <br> • Diffuse patchy infiltrates (moderate-to-severe) |
| **Tx** | **Treatment is largely supportive:** <br> Stepwise respiratory support: <br> • Keep nares clear (suction) <br> • Supplemental $O_2$ to maintain $SpO_2$ > 90-92% <br> • Heated High-Flow Nasal Cannula (HHFNC) or CPAP <br> • Invasive ventilation (priority is to allow for adequate exhalation due to hyperinflation) <br> • Consider a trial of SABA (albuterol, epinephrine) <br> • Chest physiotherapy if co-existing with neuromuscular disorder or Cystic Fibrosis <br> • Provide adequate fluids <br> • Hypertonic Solution (2015 NICE guidelines recommend against; 2014 AAP guidelines allow for administration).  It is used to increase mucociliary clearance. <br> • Use of ribavirin should be limited to severe RSV with bronchiolitis, particularly in immunocompromised children |

## BRONCHOPULMONARY DYSPLASIA (BPD)
### (NEONATAL CHRONIC LUNG DISEASE)

**Def**

Chronic lung disease associated with premature neonates who received supplemental oxygen and mechanical ventilation. This results in injury to the small airways and alveoli (including incomplete development of alveoli), reducing gas exchange surface area.

**Types**

### Diagnostic Criteria[1]

|  | < 32 weeks gestation | ≥ 32 weeks gestation |
|---|---|---|
| **Assess:** | at 36 weeks[2] | > 28 days, but < 56 days[2] |
| **Mild** | Room Air | Room Air |
| **Moderate** | FiO₂ > 21% but < 30% | FiO₂ > 21% but < 30% |
| **Severe** | FiO₂ ≥ 30% and/or Need for PPV/NCPAP | FiO₂ ≥ 30% and/or Need for PPV/NCPAP |

[1] Adapted from Jobe, A, Bancalari, E. Bronchopulmonary dysplasia. American Journal of Respiratory Critical Care Medicine, 2001.
[2] Assess at number of weeks or at discharge, whichever comes first

**Etiology**

There are many factors, including mechanical ventilation, infection, surfactant deficiency, prematurity, **oxygen toxicity**

**CM**

### *Depends on severity*
**Hallmark signs:** Hypercapnia and Hypoxemia (corrected with supplemental oxygen)
- ↓ **CL** = difficulty ventilating
- ↑ **airway obstruction** = air trapping
- **Airway hyperreactivity** (↑ risk of infections, Asthma)
- **Pulmonary Artery Hypertension (PAH)** may develop
- **Cor pulmonale** may develop

**CXR**

Varies some but diffuse haziness is common, with chronic cystic changes noted in more severe cases. Hyperinflation may be noted.

**Chronic:**
- Tracheotomy placement and long-term ventilator dependency for moderate-severe BPD
- Ventilator: Use PEEP (5-7 cm $H_2O$) to stent large airways
- Maintain compensated respiratory acidosis (normalize pH, not $PaCO_2$) with lower $V_T$ strategies
- Prophylactic treatment for RSV with palivizumab (< 2 years-old when BPD has required medical treatment within 6-months of RSV season)
- Avoid chronic use of SABA—reserve for acute exacerbation
- Avoid use of chronic steroids except infants with severe BPD who can't be weaned from ventilator and oxygen

**Acute Exacerbation:**
*May be caused by infection, airway reactivity, pulmonary edema, tube displacement*
- Closely monitor fluid status: fluid retention can quickly affect lung status (edema); consider fluid restriction
- Antibiotics should be initiated upon suspicion of infection
- Confirm tube placement
- Acute bronchospasm should be treated similarly to asthma:
  - Use of SABA (albuterol, levalbuterol)
  - Use of inhaled corticosteroids (systemic if inhaled are ineffective)
- It may be necessary to escalate ventilator settings (↑ PEEP, ↑ $FIO_2$) during an exacerbation

## BURNS (SMOKE INHALATION, THERMAL INJURY)

| | |
|---|---|
| **Def** | Inhalation of smoke, fumes, or caustic agents into the tracheo-bronchial tree with potential tissue injury due to heat or toxins. |
| **CM** | **Signs and Symptoms of Respiratory Tract Injury**<br>Facial burns, singed nasal hairs, reddened pharynx, hoarseness, cough, soot deposits, sooty sputum, central cyanosis, crackles, wheezes, stridor.  Bronchoscopy is gold standard for diagnosis.<br>$SpO_2$ can be profoundly inaccurate in the presence of increased HbCO levels - smoke inhalation.<br>**Stages**<br>Stage I – Acute respiratory distress (wheezing/stridor, ↑RR, hoarseness, cough), may occur in a few hrs,  resembles upper airway obstruction<br>Stage II – Pulmonary edema (8-36 hrs)<br>Stage III – Bacterial pneumonia (2 days – 3 weeks after injury) |
| **CXR** | **Variable:**<br>• Normal (Stage I),<br>• Pulmonary edema/ARDS (Stage II),<br>• Infiltrates (Stage III) |
| **CC** | • See **Oakes' Ventilator Management** for Mechanical Ventilation Strategies |
| **Tx** | **Begin 100% $O_2$ to all patients** (hyperbaric if CO poison), ensure adequate airway, laryngoscopy or bronchos-copy, closely monitor vitals and I&O, vigorous bronchial hygiene, bronchodilators - racemic epinephrine?, pain control?, corticosteroids?, IPV?<br><br>Burns to face, neck, oropharynx are all indicators to consider early intubation (airway swelling may not appear immediately following insult, but is likely to progress quickly once process begins)<br><br>**Treat complications:** ARDS, burns, pulmonary edema, pneumonia, respiratory failure, shock |

## CARBON MONOXIDE POISONING

**Def**

Inhalation of CO causing an inhibition of transport, delivery, and utilization of oxygen (decreased $SaO_2$ & $CaO_2$, left shift of $O_2$-Hgb curve, inhibits cytochrome c oxidase).

**Etiology**

Auto exhaust, home exhaust, space heaters, obstructed chimney, incomplete combustion of organic materials.

**CM**

**Note:** Unlike what is often heard, victims of CO poisoning are not typically "cherry red" in color. $PaO_2$ and $SpO_2$ are misleading (may appear normal but be severely hypoxic).

Symptoms vary from slight headache (COHb 10-20%) to depressed ventilation, respiratory failure, and death.

**See Oakes' Respiratory Care Pocket Guide for detailed tables and information.**

**Treatment**

Treat all victims or suspected victims of CO poisoning with 100% Oxygen (minimally nonrebreather running at 12-15 L/min) despite $SpO_2$, appearance, demeanor.

Clinical symptoms and COHb levels often do not coincide — Treat whichever is the most severe.

**Half-Life of COHb**

| In Air | 300 minutes |
|---|---|
| In 100% $O_2$ | 90 minutes |
| @ 2.5 ATA (hyperbarics) | 30 minutes |

- Monitor Cardiac, ABG's and COHb level
- Intubate and ventilate if unconscious or uncooperative
- Avoid hyperventilation and $NaHCO_3$ (shifts oxy-heme curve to left)
- Consider steroids or hypothermia
- Watch for latent deterioration (usually 4-9 days later), pulmonary edema, MI, CHF.

## PULMONARY EDEMA (CARDIOGENIC)

| | |
|---|---|
| **Def** | High pressures in the pulmonary capillaries causes a fluid shift into the alveoli and interstitium |
| **Types** | Cardiogenic – high pressure <br> Noncardiogenic – see Pediatric ARDS |
| **Etiology** | *Most Common:* Left ventricular dysfunction <br><br> *Transudation*: due to a volume/ pressure overload of the pulmonary circulation. Typical with things like fluid overload, such as with treating shock with fluid resuscitation. <br><br> *Causes*: Congenital heart disease, myocarditis, cardiomyopathy, inflammation, hypoxia, cardiac-depressant drugs. |
| **CM** | Varies with severity of underlying disorder (↑severity as ↑ fluid). <br> **General**: Sudden anxiety, restlessness, orthopnea, cyanosis, hypoxemia, diaphoresis <br> **Resp**: ↑ RR, dyspnea, cough (dry to pink, frothy fluid), basal crackles/wheezing, SOB, PND, ↓ C <br> **CV**: ↑ HR, ↓ BP, cold clammy skin, JVD, peripheral edema |
| **CXR** | **Interstitial**: Haziness of vasculature and hilar <br> **Alveolar**: Irregular, poorly defined ascinar shadows forming a "butterfly" or "bat wing" pattern. <br> **Both**: Disparity between upper and lower lobe venous calibers. LVH when due to CHF. Air-bronchograms |
| **CC** | • See **Oakes' Ventilator Management** for Mechanical Ventilation Strategies <br> • See **Oakes' Hemodynamic Monitoring** for further information on cardiopulmonary function |
| **Tx** | • Manage airway, breathing, circulation (see page 8-11) <br> • Provide noninvasive or invasive ventilator support - ensure adequate EPAP/PEEP <br> • Pharmacologic: diuretics, inotropics, afterload-reducing <br> • Reduce metabolic demand: treat fever and ↓ WOB |

## CYSTIC FIBROSIS (CF)

| | |
|---|---|
| **Def** | Genetic disease of the exocrine glands, primarily affecting the lungs, pancreas, sweat glands, and liver |
| **Types** | **Typical**<br>Sweat chloride ≥ 60 mmol<br>Disease symptoms of at least 1 organ system<br><br>**Atypical**<br>Sweat chloride not definitive (requires DNA analysis)<br>Symptoms vary |
| **Etiology** | Genetic malfunction of the cystic fibrosis transmembrane regulator (CFTR) protein leading to thickened mucus, infection, and inflammation. This may lead eventually to (severe) bronchiectasis. |
| **CM** | **Respiratory:**<br>• Persistent, productive cough<br>• Tachypnea<br>• Thick, tenacious secretions<br>• Hyperinflation of lungs (CXR, prolonged exhalation)<br>• PFT supports obstructive airway disease<br>• Digital clubbing (severe disease)<br>• Chronic colonization (*S. aureus* in children, *P. aeruginosa* in older children/adults). Repeated infections cause damage to the lungs (resulting in bronchiectasis).<br><br>**Acute Respiratory Infection:**<br>*Patients with Cystic Fibrosis quickly decompensate when exposed to a respiratory infection due to already difficult-to-manage secretions and obstructive airway disease.*<br>• ↑ cough<br>• ↑ sputum production, change in sputum<br>• ↑ tachypnea, dyspnea (at rest)<br>• ↓ FEV (PFT)<br>• CXR may or may not worsen<br>• Fever may or may not be present |

| CXR | Hyperinflation<br>Diffuse patchy infiltrates (moderate-to-severe) |
|---|---|
| Tx | **Respiratory Components of Chronic Management**<br>• CFTR Modulators (e.g. ivacaftor) - certain genotypes<br>• SABA (as a rescue treatment, and often prior to bronchial hygiene efforts, including administration of hypertonic sol)<br>• Dornase alfa (decrease viscosity of infected secretions)<br>• Hypertonic solution (hydration of secretions)<br>• Acetylcysteine (not used as often due to tendency to cause bronchospasm)<br>• Flu vaccine (inactivated form) and pneumonia vaccine are both recommended<br>• Depending on colonization, tobramycin and colistimethate may be indicated—often on an alternating schedule<br>• The use of steroids is discouraged for chronic management<br>• Chest physiotherapy is a foundation of management (either through manual CPT or using an adjunct like a vest). The goal is to develop a plan that encourages compliance.<br>• As FEV worsens (as well as 6MWT), consideration for lung transplantation (usually both lungs to avoid healthy lung from being infected by unhealthy lung by bacteria)<br><br>**Acute Infection/Hospitalization**<br>*Intermittent infections are common for most patients with CF*<br>• May consider use of systemic steroids (data varies)<br>• SABA when evidence of bronchospasm<br>• Maintain aggressive, scheduled chest physiotherapy. Strongly consider increasing frequency and duration from patient's normal schedule.<br>• As disease progresses, obstructive disease (bronchiectasis) becomes increasingly evident. Extreme caution should then be used with air trapping and accessory muscle atrophy. Use of NPPV is preferable to invasive ventilation. |

CFTR = Cystic Fibrosis Transmembrane Regulators
SABA = Short-Acting Beta Agonist
FEV = Forced Expiratory Volume
6MWT = 6-Minute Walk Test

## Cystic Fibrosis Drugs: Order of Delivery and Mixing[1]

| Therapies in Suggested Order of Administration[2] | albuterol | ipratropium | hypertonic sol | dornase alfa | tobramycin | aztreonam |
|---|---|---|---|---|---|---|
| **1. Bronchodilators (open the airways)** | | | | | | |
| albuterol | | | | | | |
| ipratropium bromide[3] | | | | | | |
| **2. Mucolytics/Mucokinetics (mobilize, thin secretions)** | | | | | | |
| hypertonic solution | | | | | | |
| dornase alfa | | | | | | |
| **3. Airway Clearance[4] - CPT, IPV, Flutter valve, etc.** | | | | | | |
| **4. Antibiotics (better deposition in infected areas)** | | | | | | |
| tobramycin | | | | | | |
| aztreonam | | | | | | |
| **5. Steroids (if indicated)[5]** | | | | | | |

[1] Green boxes have evidence to support the mixing of the drugs in the same nebulizer set-up. Red boxes indicate contraindication or lack of sufficient evidence

[2] Suggested order of administration as supported by Cystic Fibrosis Foundation, and supported by other major Cystic Fibrosis clinics

[3] Evidence is insufficient to recommend for or against long-term use

[4] Airway clearance is recommended in this order when chest physiotherapy (percussion with postural drainage) is being done. When a vest-based system is being used, it is recommended that drug delivery occur while the vest-based system is running (according to Cystic Fibrosis Foundation)

[5] Little data exists to support the use of inhaled steroids in patients with CF

| | DROWNING (FORMERLY NEAR-DROWNING) |
|---|---|
| **Def** | A process resulting in primary respiratory impairment from submersion/immersion in liquid. The victim may live (survival) or die (death by drowning) after this process. Although still used, the term *near drowning* is no longer recommended. |
| **Types** | Differences between fresh and salt water near drowning are clinically unimportant. Water temperature and the presence of contaminants in the water are greater considerations than the salinity. |
| **Etiology** | Leaving small children unattended, trauma (head/neck), exhaustion, intoxication (alcohol, drugs), seizures. |
| **CM** | Variable with minimal findings to cardiorespiratory arrest (often a delay of 2-6 hrs). **Pulmonary**: hypoxemia, SOB, tachypnea, cyanosis, pallor, crackles, frothy sputum, wheezing, cough, apnea. **Cerebral**: changed mental status, seizures, stupor, coma. **Other**: arrhythmias, evidence of trauma, metabolic acidosis, shock. |
| **CXR** | • May appear normal, especially initially<br>• Atelectasis<br>• Pulmonary edema (alveolar & interstitial infiltrates) |
| **Tx** | CPR if needed (see 2015 AHA CPR Guidelines for drowning), $O_2$ therapy ASAP (maintain $SpO_2$ > 94%), treat bronchospasm, treat hypothermia if present, treat respiratory failure with $O_2$, NPPV, MV with PEEP, (treat ARDS). Use PEEP early (especially if $O_2$ > 40%).<br>Treat cerebral edema with diuretics<br>Treat pulmonary edema ("secondary drowning") with diuretics and PEEP/CPAP. Watch for arrhythmias, inotropic drugs to improve tissue and cerebral perfusion? Antibiotics? (If infected source). |

# INTRACRANIAL PRESSURE (ICP)

**Def**

ICP is the pressure of cerebral spinal fluid in the cerebral ventricles, which is determined by both CSF circulation and cerebral blood flow. Excessive pressure results in pressure against the brain with particular concern for brain herniation.

**Etiology**

**Causes of Intracranial Hypertension:**
- Traumatic brain injury (TBI) is most common cause
- Hydrocephalus/Hypertensive encephalopathy
- Tumor (CNS)
- Infections (encephalitis, meningitis, abscess)

**CM**

**Measurement of ICP and CPP in Pediatrics**
  *Intracranial Pressure (ICP)*
  ICP > 20 mm Hg (for > 5 mins) requires treatment
  **Normal ICP by Age**

| Infants | 1.5-6 mm Hg |
|---|---|
| Children | 3-7 mm Hg |
| Adolescents | < 10-15 mm Hg |

  **Cerebral Perfusion Pressure (CPP)**
  normal (mm Hg): 0-5 yrs = 40-50; 6-17 yrs = 50-60

**Acute ↑ ICP:**
- Irregular respiratory pattern or apnea
- ↑ mean arterial pressure (MAP)
- Headache/double or blurry vision
- Vomiting
- Δ Mental status
- Seizures (some types)

**Symptoms of Impending Brain Herniation:**
- Irregular respiratory pattern or apnea
- Bradycardia
- Hypertension
- Pupils unequal, dilated, unresponsive
- Posturing (decorticate, decerebrate)

**Hypertension + bradycardia + irregular respiratory pattern =**
Cushing triad (late signs of impending herniation)
*Children may be tachycardic instead of bradycardic (PALS)*

**Tx**

**GOAL**: Minimize ICP and Maintain CPP
- Ensure adequate support of airway, breathing, circulation
- Ensure head is midline, spine is stabilized if trauma is suspected (PALS)
- Intubate when GCS ≤ 8 (or declining rapidly in general); inability to protect airway, insufficient respiratory drive, or with acute herniation (due to need to hyperventilate)
- Maintain normal ABGs
  - Hypoxemia results in vasodilation which may ↑ ICP
  - Hypercapnia results in vasodilation which may ↑ ICP
- Elevate head 15-30 degrees, keep midline (allows for maximum venous return from head)
- Avoid fever (use cooling blankets, antipyretics)
- Control pain/agitation aggressively (PALS)
- Drugs: Consider management of ↑ ICP
- Ventilator: use extreme caution with high PIP or PEEP (may ↓ venous drainage from head)

**Important Note on Hyperventilating (PALS)**

Do NOT use PaCO₂ < 30 mm Hg to prophylactically treat ↑ ICP. This may result in ↓ cardiac output, as well as cerebral vasoconstriction (brain ischemia and worse outcomes)

Very cautiously consider MILD hyperventilation (PaCO₂ > 30 mm Hg) in the initial 48-hours after injury. *Use should be a rare rescue adjunct.*

# PEDIATRIC ACUTE RESPIRATORY DISTRESS SYNDROME (PARDS OR PEDIATRIC ARDS)

An acute, diffuse, inflammatory lung injury resulting in diminished FRC, severe shunting, alveolar transudates, ↓ surfactant (washout) atelectasis, ↓ compliance, and severe hypoxemia.

*This topic reflects the Pediatric Acute Lung Injury Consensus Conference (PALICC) and Pediatric Advanced Life Support (PALS).*

## Diagnostic Criteria:

Exclusion: patients with perinatal-related lung disease

### 1. Acute Onset of Respiratory Distress

*Must be within 7 days of a defined event (sepsis, trauma, pneumonia, etc.). Most cases occur within 72 hours.*

### 2. Hypoxemia:

| Noninvasive Support (use P/F or S/F) | | |
|---|---|---|
| *Patient is on BiPAP (full face mask) or CPAP ≥ 5 cm H₂O)* | | |
| P/F ratio | ≤ **300** | $PaO_2/FiO_2$ |
| S/F ratio | ≤ **264** | $SpO_2/FiO_2$ |

| Invasive Support (use OI unless PaO₂ unavailable) | | | |
|---|---|---|---|
| Mild | OI | 4 ≤ OI < 8 | $(FiO_2 \times mPAW \times 100)/PaO_2$ |
| | OSI | 5 ≤ OSI < 7.5 | $(FiO_2 \times mPAW \times 100)/SpO_2$ |
| Moderate | OI | 8 ≤ OI < 16 | $(FiO_2 \times mPAW \times 100)/PaO_2$ |
| | OSI | 7.5 ≤ OSI < 12.3 | $(FiO_2 \times mPAW \times 100)/SpO_2$ |
| Severe | OI | OI ≥ 16 | $(FiO_2 \times mPAW \times 100)/PaO_2$ |
| | OSI | OSI ≥ 12.3 | $(FiO_2 \times mPAW \times 100)/SpO_2$ |

*OI = Oxygenation Index; OSI = Oxygen Saturation Index.*
*FiO₂ should be entered into the equations as a decimal, not a percent*

## Patients at risk of PARDS    minimum flow or FiO₂:

| O₂ via mask, nasal cannula, or high flow | < 1 yr: 2 L/min        1-5 yrs: 4 L/min<br>5-10 yrs: 6 L/min    > 10 yrs: 8 L/min |
|---|---|
| Nasal mask CPAP or BiPAP | FiO₂ ≤ 40%<br>(to maintain SpO₂ 88-97%) |
| Invasive Ventilation | FiO₂ to keep SpO₂ ≤ 88%<br>(with OI > 4 or OSI > 5) |

**Def (cont.)**

**3. Bilateral consolidation on CXR or CT**
Evidence of new infiltrates consistent with acute pulmonary parenchymal disease (even if unilateral)

**4. Ruled out cardiac failure and fluid overload**
Left ventricular failure and fluid overload should be ruled out, but patients with heart disease are not ruled out

**Etiology**

| Respiratory (Direct) | Non-Respiratory (Indirect) |
|---|---|
| • **Aspiration** (gastric especially) | • **Sepsis** (most common cause) |
| • Foreign body obstruction | • Blood transfusion reactions |
| • Drowning injuries | (transfusion-related acute |
| • $O_2$ toxicity | lung injury) |
| • Pneumonia (all types) | • Burns (massive) |
| • Raised ICP (head injury) | • DIC |
| • Smoke inhalation | • Drugs/Alcohol poisoning or |
| • Thoracic irradiation | overdose |
| • Thoracic trauma | • Fat embolism |
| • Ventilator-induced injury | • Malignancy |
| | • Shock (severe, prolonged) |

## Phases
*(there is often overlap in the phases; this is a rough guide)*

Phase 1 (first 7-10 days) Exudative
*Intense inflammatory response, resulting in:*
• Alveolar and endothelial damage
• Increased vascular permeability = pulmonary edema
• Increased water and protein
• Some component of pulmonary hypertension

Phase 2 (10+ days) Fibroproliferative
*Extensive pulmonary fibrosis, which usually resolves
(acute fibrosis resolves, some fibrosis may remain)*

**Initial phase is marked by refractory hypoxemia, requiring a high amount of supplemental oxygen.**
**After the first few days, the O₂ requirement may decrease.**

| General | • Agitated, anxious, confused, restless<br>• Rapid-onset (usually within 72 hrs) |
|---|---|
| Respiratory | • Palpation |
| Pulm. Dyn | • ↓ CL (total C < 30 mL/cm $H_2O$)<br>• ↑PIP (vent)<br>• ↓TC; ↑$\dot{V}$D |
| ABG's | • **Oxygenation** – refractory hypoxemia ($PaO_2/FIO_2$ ≤300), ↑ shunt (> 20%)<br>• Ventilation – respiratory alkalosis → respiratory acidosis |
| Cardiovasc. | • ↑ HR<br>• PCWP < 15-18 mm Hg*<br>• PAD – PCWP > 5mmHg |

*Compare with CHF: PCWP > 15-18 mm Hg.*

**2-24 hrs**: Bilateral opacities (diffuse or not) and interstitial infiltrates (peripheral and dependent zones), air bronchograms.*
**24-48 hrs**: coalesce to produce massive air space consolidation in both lungs.
* Compare with CHF: cardiomegaly, perihilar infiltrates, pleural effusion.

• Pediatric Acute Lung Injury Consensus. Pediatric Critical Care Medicine 2015.
• The ARDS Definition Task Force. Acute Respiratory Distress Syndrome: The Berlin Definition. JAMA 2012.

**General Considerations:**
- The goals are to provide supportive care, prevent further injury (to the lungs and elsewhere), and maintain adequate (not normal) oxygenation
- Supplemental oxygen alone may not help (due to the refractory nature of ARDS), so should be used in conjunction with CPAP/PEEP strategies.
- Drugs (Analgesics and Sedation) may increase synchrony with the ventilator and ↓ $O_2$ consumption. Paralytics may need to be considered when pain/sedation is inadequate in allowing for adequate ventilation
- Hemodynamic monitoring:
  - Arterial line (hemodynamics and ABG draws)
  - Central line (hemodynamics and drug access)
  - Pulmonary artery line (hemodynamics—less common)
- Consider RBC transfusion when Hgb < 7.0 g/dL
- Careful fluid management has been shown to improve outcomes (Goal of CVP < ~4 mm Hg)
- Use of inflated, cuffed ET Tube is recommended (may allow leak in HFOV to improve $CO_2$ elimination)

Tx

**Oxygenation/Ventilation Goals**

| $O_2$ | *Optimize PEEP (see next page), then:* |
|---|---|
| | <u>PARDS with PEEP < 10 cm $H_2O$:</u><br>Keep $SpO_2$ 92-97%<br><br><u>PARDS with PEEP > 10 cm $H_2O$:</u><br>Keep $SpO_2$ 88-92%<br>Monitor central venous saturation |
| $CO_2$ | <u>Moderate-to-Severe PARDS:</u><br>Permissive hypercapnia (pH 7.15-7.30)<br><br>*Exceptions*: ↑ ICP, severe pulmonary hypertension, hemodynamic instabilitiy, significant ventricular dysfunction |
| $NaHCO_3$ | Sodium bicarbonate administration is not generally recommended |

## Ventilator Strategies

| VT | Based on pathophysiology/compliance: 5-8 mL/kg, drop to 3-6 mL/kg if ↓ CL |
|---|---|
| Pplat | Keep 28 cm $H_2O$ or below<br>May consider 29-32 cm $H_2O$ in certain circumstances (↓ CL) |
| PEEP | Titrate to oxygen goals<br>Carefully monitor hemodynamic status, compliance: 10-15 cm $H_2O$<br>Severe PARDS: > 15 cm $H_2O$<br>Recruitment Maneuvers: Consider slow incremental and decremental steps instead of sustained inflation |
| High-Frequency | <u>HFOV</u>: Use when Pplat > 28 cm $H_2O$ (unless known ↓ chest wall compliance). Titrate MAP for recruitment as $O_2$, $CO_2$, hemodynamics are monitored<br><u>HFJV</u>: Consider possible for severe air leak syndrome<br><u>HFPPV</u>: Consider possibly if secretion-induced atelectasis |

iNO is not recommended routinely, but may be considered in patients with pulmonary hypertension or severe right ventricular dysfunction.

### Noninvasive Ventilation (NPPV)

- Consider for children at risk of PARDS, particularly those at greater risk of complications from invasive ventilation (immunodeficiency, for example)
- NPPV should be seen as a trial. If there is no clinical improvement, invasive ventilation should be considered
- High-flow nasal cannula is not an equal substitution for NPPV

### Extracorporeal Membrane Oxygenation (ECMO)

- Consider case-by-case with severe PARDS when the respiratory failure is likely to be reversible, or child is a candidate for lung transplantation

| | PEDIATRIC CHEST TRAUMA |
|---|---|
| **Types** | See Table on following pages for specific trauma types typically found with children |
| **Etiology** | **Trauma varies in pediatrics:**<br>• Chest wall compliance (greater in children) which may result in serious internal injuries with no notable damage to the chest wall, as well as direct traumas to the heart<br>• The mediastinum is more mobile in children, resulting in more of a mediastinal shift, resulting in ↓ CO, ↓ BP<br>• Children deteriorate (transition from respiratory distress to failure) quickly, at least partially due to metabolic demands |
| **CM** | **Specific clinical manifestations are on the following pages.**<br><br>**General findings that suggest chest trauma:**<br>• Respiratory distress (nasal flaring, retractions, etc.)<br>• Respiratory rate (increased, may be decreased)<br>• Crepitus, tenderness, physical signs like bruising<br>• Abnormal breath sounds<br>• Paradoxical chest wall movement<br>• Jugular venous distension (JVD)<br><br>**Immediate considerations:** ECG, Imaging (CXR), Labs |
| **CXR** | **See tables on next pages for CXR considerations** |
| **Tx** | Perform rapid assessment with particular focus on Airway, Breathing, Circulation. See Pediatric Resuscitation (Ch 8) for details. Specific suggestions are on the following pages by type of trauma.<br><br>During initial assessment, support by ensuring patent airway adequate oxygenation and ventilation.<br><br>Do not delay critical interventions (needle thoracostomy, pericardiocentesis) |

# Thoracic Trauma Types: Signs, Treatments, Complications

| Injury | Signs and Symptoms | Possible Treatments | Complications |
|---|---|---|---|
| Rib Fractures | Dyspnea<br>Chest pain/point tenderness<br>Tachypnea<br>Tachycardia | Pain control<br>Deep breathing exercises<br>Treat complications | Pneumothorax<br>Hemothorax<br>Underlying internal injury<br>Atelectasis (shallow breaths) |
| Flail chest (same as rib fractures +) | ↑ Dyspnea<br>Paradoxical respirations (if no PPV)<br>Mediastinal shift (possible)<br>Cyanosis | Stabilize injury or positive pressure ventiation | Atelectasis<br>Shock<br>Respiratory failure |
| Pneumothorax | See Air Leak Syndromes - Page 3-5 | | |
| Hemothorax | > 25% blood volume lost:<br>Restlessness/anxiety<br>**Hypotension**<br>Mediastinal shift (possible) | Chest tube placement<br>*immediate if distress/shock* | Hypovolemic shock<br>Pulmonary contusion<br>Respiratory failure |
| Cardiac Tamponade | Jugular venous distension<br>Hypotension<br>Tachycardia<br>(if bradycardia, arrest is imminent)<br>Narrowed pulse pressure | **Acute = Life-Threatening**<br>Pericardiocentesis<br>Surgical interventions<br>Fluid resuscitation<br>Inotropes | Hypovolemic shock<br>Cardiogenic shock<br>PPV may ↓ CO further |

| Injury | Signs and Symptoms | Possible Treatments | Complications |
|--------|--------------------|--------------------|---------------|
| Pulmonary Contusion<br><br>(Diagnosed by history of chest trauma + any of the bold items) | (asymptomatic-to-severe symptoms)<br>**Tachypnea**<br>**Hypoxemia**<br>**Abnormal breath sounds**<br>Dyspnea<br>Cyanosis<br>Tachycardia<br>Hypotension<br>CXR: consolidation | Support oxygenation and ventilation (consider NPPV) | Respiratory failure<br>Pneumonia |
| Diaphragmatic Rupture | (asymptomatic-to-severe symptoms)<br>Dyspnea<br>Nausea/Vomiting<br>Pain (abdominal, chest)<br>Tachycardia<br>Tachypnea<br>Abdomen is scaphoid or distended<br>↓ breath sounds (ipsilateral)<br>Bowel sounds in chest<br>CXR: ↑ diaphragm, bowel in chest, signs of atelectasis | Nasogastric tube to decompress stomach (children are likely to gulp air)<br>Treat respiratory distress<br>Surgical interventions<br>Avoid chest tube placement (may injure displaced organs) | Bowel obstruction |

| Injury | Signs and Symptoms | Possible Treatments | Complications |
|--------|--------------------|--------------------|---------------|
| **Myocardial Contusion** | Persistent unexplained tachycardia<br>Chest pain/tenderness<br>Tachypnea<br>Murmur<br>Crackles (late) | Pain control | ↓ Cardiac output<br>Arrhythmias<br>Cardiac arrest/shock<br>Cardiac tamponade |
| **Traumatic Aortic Injury** | Retrosternal or interscapular pain<br>Dyspnea<br>Stridor<br>Dysphagia<br>Hypertension<br>CXR: widened mediastinum, aortic knob blurring, left pleural effusion | Immediate surgical consult | Hypovolemic shock<br>Death |

## SHOCK

**Def**

Inadequate tissue perfusion resulting in hypoxic insult and causing widespread abnormal cell metabolism and membrane dysfunction.

**Types**

### Hypovolemic Shock
↓ effective circulating volume (most common)

### Distributive/Vasodilatory Shocks
(↓ SVR, abnormal blood distribution, poor tissue perfusion)
**Septic** (most common distributive shock in children) –
Relative hypovolemia caused by any infection.
**Anaphylactic** – Systemic allergic reaction causing circulatory failure
**Neurogenic** – Sympathetic nervous system dysfunction resulting in massive peripheral vasodilation or hypoperfusion

### Cardiogenic Shock
Systemic hypoperfusion due to heart failure

### Obstructive Shock
Impaired cardiac output as a result of blood flow being obstructed. Includes cardiac tamponade, tension pneumothorax, and massive pulmonary embolism

**Etiology**

### Stages
**Compensated Shock:** the body is able to maintain adequate perfusion (there is a normal blood pressure)
**Decompensated Shock:** the body is no longer able to maintain adequate perfusion to vital organs (hypotension is now present)
**Irreversible Shock:** Irreversible organ damage and death occurs. Prognosis is poor.

See Oakes' Hemodynamic Monitoring Pocket Guide for comprehensive information on Shocks

## Causes

**Hypovolemia:** bleeding, vomiting or diarrhea

**Cardiogenic:**

Trauma (aneurysm, septal defects, ruptures,
tension pneumothorax or pneumopericardium)

Congenital (see congenital heart diseases)

Dysrhythmias (see Pediatric Resuscitation chapter)

Metabolic (acidosis, hypocalcemia, hyperkalemia)

Ischemic (myocardial infarction, Kawasaki disease)

**Sepsis:** fever, known infection

### Critical Signs & Symptoms to Monitor

| Sign/Symptom | Compensated | Decompensated |
|---|---|---|
| **Blood Pressure** | BP Normal | ↓ (late finding) |
| **Heart Rate** | ↑ | ↑↑ |
| **Respiratory Rate** | ↑ | ↑↑ or ↓ |
| **Respiratory Pattern** | Rapid, Shallow | Labored, Irregular |
| **Central pulse** | Usually normal | Weakening |
| **Peripheral pulse** | Normal or ↓ | ↓↓ or absent |
| **Pulse pressure** | Normal or ↓ | Narrowing |
| **Extremities** | Warm | Cool |
| **Capillary Refill** | Normal | Prolonged |
| **Level of Consciousness** | Normal or Altered | Decreased |

Once a child is hypotensive, organ perfusion is likely
compromised. It is critical to intervene before
compensated shock becomes decompensated.

**Other signs and symptoms** are dependent on type and
severity of shock, but include:

- Diaphoresis
- Agitation/fussiness/confusion
- Skin appears gray, dusky, or cyanotic
- Decreased urine output
- Malaise or poor feeding

CM

## Summary of PALS recommendations:

**Position**
- If responsive, allow child to be comfortable
- If unresponsive, hypotensive, but breathing well, place in supine position

**Respiratory:**
- Give adequate oxygen to all children in shock.
- High-flow is preferred, but NPPV or invasive mechanical ventilation may be necessary

**Vascular Access:**
- Stabilize airway/breathing, then gain vascular access
- Compensated: peripheral is acceptable
- Hypotensive: Immediate access is needed (even if IO)

**Fluid Resuscitation:**
- General: Isotonic crystalloid 20 mL/kg over 5-20 mins
- If severe, hypotensive, hypovolemic: give over 5-10 min
- If cardiogenic shock: 5-10 mL/kg over 10-20 minutes. Carefully monitor (stop if pulm. edema or ↓ tissue perfusion)
- Reassess and repeat 20 mL/kg until adequate BP/perfusion

**Monitoring: Positive Response Indicators**

| SpO₂ | ≥ 94% |
|---|---|
| HR | Toward Normal |
| Peripheral Pulse | Weaker → Stronger <br> Bounding → ↓, but strong |
| Cap Refill | Shorten |
| Skin Color | Normal |
| Skin Temp | Warmer |
| Blood Pressure | ↑ to Normal Range <br> (normal pulse pressure) |
| LOC | ↑ Responsiveness |
| Fluid Loss | Vomiting/diarrhea controlled |
| Urine Output | Inf/Child: ~1.5-2 mL/kg/hr <br> Child/Adoles.: ~ 1 mL/kg/hr |

Tx

## Monitor Laboratory Values
### Selected Abnormal Findings, Causes, and Strategies

| | |
|---|---|
| ↓ Hgb/Hct | Hemorrhage? Dilution? Hemolysis?<br>Give 100% $O_2$<br>Control bleeding/Blood transfusion<br>Monitor fluid resuscitation |
| ↑↓ WBC | ? Sepsis<br>Obtain cultures/give antibiotics |
| ↓ Platelets | DIC? ↓ platelet production?<br>Transfuse platelets (if serious bleeding) |
| ↑↓ Glucose | Stress? Sepsis? ↓ production?<br>Treat if ↑ or ↓ |
| ↑↓ Potassium | Acidosis? Diuresis? Renal?<br>Treat if significant ↑ or ↓<br>Correct acidosis |
| ↓ Calcium | Sepsis? Transfusion? Colloid? Bicarb?<br>Give calcium |
| ↑ BUN, Creatinine | Indicator of renal perfusion<br>Dopamine? IV fluids with diuretics? |
| ↑ Lactate | Hypoxia? ↑ Glucose? ↓ Metabolism?<br>Treat acidosis; Improve perfusion |
| ABG | Evaluate ABG<br>Treat as indicated (many causes)<br>Evaluate anion gap |
| ScvO₂ | ↓ indicates inadequate $O_2$ delivery or<br>   ↑ $O_2$ consumption<br>↑ indicates blood flow maldistribution or<br>   ↓ $O_2$ utilization<br>Goal: ↑ $O_2$ delivery, ↓ $O_2$ demand |

DIC: Disseminated intravascular coagulation

### Drug Therapy (see Pediatric Resuscitation for Details)
Goal: affect contractility, rate, and vascular resistance
  Inotropes (Dopamine, Epinephrine, Dobutamine)
  Phosphodiesterase Inhibitors (Milrinone)
  Vasodilators (Nitroglycerin, Nitroprusside)
  Vasopressors (Epinephrine, Norepinephrine,
           Dopamine, Vasopressin)

## UPPER AIRWAY OBSTRUCTIONS

| Types | Acute epiglottitis (*Haemophilus influenza Type B*)<br>Croup (laryngotracheobronchitis-parainfluenza)<br>Foreign Body Airway Obstruction (see page 8-7) |
|---|---|
| CM | *While rare, epiglottitis is a life-threatening emergency and should still be considered in assessing a child* |

|  | Epiglottitis | Croup |
|---|---|---|
| **Age** | > 3 years | < 3 years |
| **Progression** | Rapid (4-12 hrs) | Gradual (> 24 hrs)<br>may follow URI |
| **Position** | Sitting, Leaning forward | Any position |
| **Swallow** | Drooling, Sore throat | No drooling (swallow) |
| **Voice** | Muffled | Hoarse |
| **Anxiety** | Anxious | Unlikely to be anxious |
| **Fever** | > 39° C (↑ WBC) | < 39° C (normal WBC) |
| **Throat** | Red, inflamed | Mildly red, swollen |
| **Respiratory Distress** | | |
| **Stridor** | Marked inspiratory | Mild inspiratory +<br>expiratory |
| **Cough** | None | Barking, Brassy |
| **Breath Sounds** | ↓ | ↓ |
| **Retractions** | Maybe | Maybe |
| **CXR** | Thumb sign | Steeple sign |
| **Treatments** | | |
| **Critical Steps** | Do NOT agitate<br>**Emergent intubation**[1]<br>Treat as critically<br>difficult airway | Minimize agitation<br>Racemic epinephrine<br>Cool aerosol |

[1] Carefully prepare for intubation. Transport to OR for intubation should be considered. Do not visualize epiglottitis until immediately ready to intubate. Airway management is critical.

## VIRAL INFECTIONS (INFLUENZAS, PNEUMONIAS)

| | |
|---|---|
| **Def** | Acute respiratory tract viral infection characterized by the sudden onset of symptoms. |
| **Etiology** | There is a wide variety of viruses responsible for infection. Infections in general can be viral, bacterial, or fungal. Viral is the most common, but since there is no effective treatment for most viruses, the goal is supportive care<br><br>*Typical viruses:*<br>Croup (see Upper Airway Obstructions)<br>Influenzas (flu)<br>Pneumonia (some are bacterial)<br>Pneumonitis (chemical, infectious, aspiration)<br>Respiratory Synctial Virus (see RSV)<br>Rhinovirus (common cold) |
| **CM** | Symptoms vary by severity of infection and amount of respiratory involvement.<br>See respiratory distress symptoms (page 9-6) for further details |
| **Tx** | Because this is viral, only limited options are available (which slow the progression, decreasing severity and length of the illness).<br><br>Respiratory goals are to provide supportive care. It is important to remember that children decompensate quickly in response to respiratory distress. Identifying early signs and symptoms of respiratory distress are critical in providing preventative measures to respiratory failure.<br><br>• Watch for congestion. Infants are obligate nose breathers until 3-6 months old (at which point they may still prefer nasal breathing). Maintaining patent nares (bulb suction) is important.<br>• Support oxygenation: supplemental $O_2$, etc.<br>• Support ventilation: noninvasively or invasively<br>• Treat bronchospasm: MDI or SVN albuterol<br>• Support bronchial hygiene: suctioning, CPT, hypertonic?<br>• Treat infection (bacterial): start antibiotics within an hour |

CONTENTS

Pediatric

Ventilation

CONTENTS

## Some Notes About This Chapter

**Terms/Abbreviations Used**

| mPAW | **Mean Airway Pressure** We have decided on this abbreviation as it is easy to differentiate from any other abbreviation. Other acceptable abbreviations include MAP (also Mean Arterial Pressure), P̄aw, Pa̅w. |
|------|---|
| FIO₂ | **Oxygen Percentage** $FIO_2$ by definition is a decimal equivalent of the fractional inspired oxygen. It is more clinically relevant to set $O_2$ by %, so you will see $FIO_2$ used as a % in this chapter. |

**Special Note:**

This chapter presents some basic concepts and guidelines. Pediatric ventilation settings should be carefully considered in the context of pathophysiology and clinical condition.

*For detailed Noninvasive and Invasive Mechanical Ventilation Strategies, including:*
- Graphic Interpretation
- Equations
- Troubleshooting
- Additional Modes of Ventilation

*See*
**Oakes' Ventilator Management Pocket Guide**

→

*available at RespiratoryBooks.com*

## ■ General Considerations

### Pediatric Anatomy/Physiology Affecting Ventilation

| Anatomy | Infant | Growth | Adult |
|---------|--------|--------|-------|
| Tongue | Large | $\longrightarrow\longrightarrow$ | Normal |
| Epiglottis shape | Floppy Omega-shaped | $\longrightarrow\longrightarrow$ | Firm Flat |
| Epiglottis level | C3 - C4 | $\longrightarrow\longrightarrow$ | C5 - C6 |
| Trachea | Small Short | $\longrightarrow\longrightarrow$ | Wide Long |
| Larynx shape | Funnel-shaped | $\longrightarrow\longrightarrow$ | Columnar |
| Narrowest point | subglottic | $\longrightarrow\longrightarrow$ | level of vocal cords |
| Lung volumes | ~250 mL at birth | $\longrightarrow\longrightarrow$ | ~6000 mL |
| Compliance | greater compliance of trachea, larynx, bronchi | $\longrightarrow\longrightarrow$ | lesser compliance of trachea, larynx, bronchi (due to cartilage) |

*Anatomical and physiological maturity occurs gradually, and not all changes occur at the same rate.*

# ■ Monitoring

*Use all monitoring techniques in the context of careful systematic evaluation and critical thinking.*

**SEE ALSO: Pediatric Assessment Chapter**

**Continuous Monitoring:**
- Cardiac activity (monitor—including HR)
- Carbon dioxide (TcCO$_2$, ETCO$_2$)
- Oxygen delivery (SpO$_2$)
- Proximal airway pressures (PIP, PEEP, mPAW)
- Respiratory Rate
- Tidal Volume (VT) delivery
- I:E ratio ($f$, TI, etc.)

**Periodic Monitoring:**
- Acid-Base (CBG, VBG, ABG)
- Blood Pressure (invasive or noninvasive)
- Chest X-Ray
- Endotracheal tube position and cuff pressure (if cuffed)
- Physical assessment (auscultation, WOB, etc.)
- Ventilator/patient trends
  - Airway compliance (Cstat, Cdyn)
  - Airway resistance (PIP, Raw)
  - Synchrony (patient appearance and graphics)

# ■ Noninvasive and Invasive Parameters

**Conventional Ventilator Parameters Overview**
*(more detailed information can be found later in this chapter)*

| Parameter | Average Normal Settings |
|---|---|
| Peak Inspiratory Pressure (PIP) | 15-25 cm $H_2O$ |
| Tidal Volume (VT) | ~6 mL/kg IBW *(lung protection)*<br>6-10 mL/kg IBW *(normal)* |
| Positive End Expiratory Pressure (PEEP) | 4-7 cm $H_2O$ |
| Frequency (*f*) or Rate | ~ age appropriate RR |
| I:E Ratio | 1:1 to 1:3 |
| Inspiratory Time (TI) | Varies by age/RR |
| Flow Waveform | Decelerating  Square  Sinusoidal |
| FIO$_2$ (O$_2$%) | 21% - 100%<br>(< 50% when possible) |

## Tidal Volume (VT)

| Usual Range | | |
|---|---|---|
| | Infant | 5-6 mL/kg |
| | Toddler | 5-8 mL/kg |
| | Child | 6-10 mL/kg |
| | Adolescent | 6-10 mL/kg IBW |

**OR:**
(average initial setting for all age groups):
- ~6 mL/kg IBW for lung protection
- 6-10 mL/kg IBW for normal lungs

| Clinical Notes | *In the absence of VT measurement, aim for a gentle rise and fall of the chest.* |
|---|---|

- In pressure-controlled modes, VT is an indicator of changing lung dynamics (compliance, resistance)
- In pressure-controlled modes, set inspiratory pressure is usually titrated to ensure a safe tidal volume range (see Normal Range above)

| Cautions | |
|---|---|

- Most clinicians favor a tidal volume in the lower part of the appropriate range to avoid volutrauma. There are exceptions to this (such as neuromuscular disorders).
- Tidal volume measurements in small infants are particularly vulnerable to compressible volume of gas in the ventilator circuit. Measuring tidal volume delivery at the endotracheal tube/vent circuit connection is preferred.

Pediatric

Ventilation

| Peak Inspiratory Pressure (PIP) | |
|---|---|
| **Average Range** | 15-25 cm $H_2O$<br>(maintain < 30 cm $H_2O$) |
| **Clinical Notes** | The lowest PIP that adequately ventilates the patient is usually appropriate<br>To recruit alveoli, appropriate PEEP is crucial<br>PIP should remain < 30 cm $H_2O$ in infants and children and higher PIPs should be avoided, if possible, but may be necessary in some patients with HCL<br>When high PIPs are used to open closed alveoli, the open alveoli may over-distend, resulting in volutrauma |
| **Cautions** | Rapidly changing (increasing) $C_L$ and FRC places the patient at high risk for lung over-distension and resultant air leaks. $V_T$ should be continuously monitored.<br>It is critically important to understand the difference between ventilators that are PEEP-compensated and ones that are not (see caution below) |
| **Selecting Initial PIP** | PIP is set in pressure modes:<br>1. Adjust PIP to a target tidal volume range<br>2. Use the Pressure-Volume Loop: adjust PIP until there is little/no flattening of the loop |

**Caution**: Some ventilators (and some models of the same ventilator) define PIP differently.
**PEEP-compensated**: baseline is the set PEEP (adds PIP to PEEP)
**not-PEEP-compensated**: baseline is ZERO for each

| Type | PEEP-compensated | Not-PEEP-compensated |
|---|---|---|
| (Peak) Inspiratory Pressure | 15 | 15 |
| PEEP | 5 | 5 |
| Delta-P | 20 | 10 |

11-8

| Mean Airway Pressure (mPAW) | |
|---|---|
| **Normal Range** | 5-15 cm $H_2O$ |
| **Clinical Notes** | **mPAW** is often the most critical factor in determining optimal oxygenation as it correlates with lung volume. Generally, there is a linear rise in mean $PaO_2$ with ↑ mPAW until over-distension occurs, then a ↓ $PaO_2$ (and ↑ $PaCO_2$) occurs.<br>*Factors affecting mPAW (in probable order of magnitude):* PEEP, TI, PIP/VT, $f$ (↓TE), VI, and pressure waveform (see diagram below)<br><br>**Approximation of mPAW:**<br>$$mPAW = \frac{\left[\dfrac{(PIP \times TI)}{Total\ Cycle\ Time} + (PEEP \times TE)\right]}{Total\ Cycle\ Time}$$<br>*Optimal level:* The lowest level in which gas exchange is most efficient and beyond which alveolar over-distension occurs |

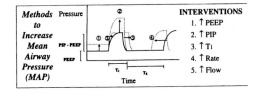

| Methods to Increase Mean Airway Pressure (MAP) | Pressure | **INTERVENTIONS** |
|---|---|---|

**INTERVENTIONS**
1. ↑ PEEP
2. ↑ PIP
3. ↑ TI
4. ↑ Rate
5. ↑ Flow

| Positive End Expiratory Pressure (PEEP) | |
|---|---|
| Usual Range | 4-7 cm $H_2O$<br>(maintain open-lung approach without causing hemodynamic compromise) |
| Clinical Notes | PEEP is used to prevent airway/alveolar collapse and establish functional residual capacity (FRC).<br>Maintaining open lungs is highly preferred over atelectrauma (caused by opening and closing of collapsed alveoli)<br>Primarily used to improve oxygenation ($\uparrow$ FRC), but recruited lung units may improve V/Q, thus improving ventilation secondarily |
| Selecting Initial PEEP | ~5 cm $H_2O$ |
| Optimal PEEP | 1. Use P-V loop (approximately 2-3 cm $H_2O$ above the lower inflection point) to set PEEP, allow for recruitment, and then wean using P-V loop<br>2. Incremental PEEP (increase PEEP, monitor change in VT with close watch of hemodynamics)<br>3. PEEP/$FiO_2$ tables are not recommended as they were developed in the adult population |
| Monitoring | Increase in $PaO_2$<br>CXR: monitor under/over expansion<br>P-V Loop: shift of PIP down at same VT (remember VT should be set) |
| Complications | $\downarrow$ venous return, barotrauma<br>(too much PEEP results in overdistension) |

| Frequency (f) or Rate | | |
|---|---|---|
| Normal Range | Infant | 25-40 breaths/min |
| | Toddler | 20-35 breaths/min |
| | Child | 18-30 breaths/min |
| | Adolescent | 12-20 breaths/min |
| Clinical Notes | Used most commonly to adjust $PaCO_2$ and pH<br>General rule of thumb: ↓ CL requires ↑ f<br>The rate should be set in context of disease state, child's age, and clinical response<br>Adequacy of rate can be assessed by physical assessment, pH/$PaCO_2$ | |
| Cautions | High rates = ↓ TE and may lead to air-trapping with inadvertent PEEP, and ↓ venous return and ↓ CO | |

Pediatric

Ventilation

| Inspiratory Time (TI) | | |
|---|---|---|
| **Normal Range** | Infant | 0.4-0.5 sec |
| | Toddler | 0.6-0.7 sec |
| | Child | 0.6-0.75 sec |
| | Adolescent | 0.7-1.0 sec |
| **Clinical Notes** | Select TI for patient comfort and synchronous breathing. Considerations include lung time constants, patient age, and breathing pattern. | |

| ↓ CL | short TC | Use short TI |
|---|---|---|
| ↑ Raw | Long TC | Use long TI |

TC = Time Constant

| **Cautions** | TI is usually not set below 0.4 sec in PICU The longer the TI (especially > 1.0 sec), the greater the risk of barotrauma, adverse cardiac effects. Carefully observe flow waveforms to ensure exhalation to baseline Longer TI = ↓ TE (assuming same rate) |
|---|---|

## STUDENT tip

Remember that neonates, infants, and young children can have significantly higher respiratory rates. This will result in a much shorter Total Cycle Time (TCT = $60/f$), which decreases inspiratory time and then available expiratory time.

| Inspiratory Flow ($\dot{V}I$) | |
|---|---|
| **Clinical Notes** | **Volume Ventilation** (if able to set):<br>set to lowest value that will generate the desired PIP/Pressure waveform<br>Minimum flow should be 2x $\dot{V}E$. Ideal $\dot{V}I =$ 3 x $\dot{V}E$.<br>High flows may be needed to maintain VT when TI is shortened. Flows > 10 L/min may result in ↓ VT due to ↑ turbulence in small ET Tubes and ↑ risk of air-leaks.<br>Slower $\dot{V}Is$ are used for patients with ↑ Raw and/or poor gas distribution<br><br>**Pressure Ventilation**: Flow is determined by patient characteristics |
| **Cautions** | **Signs of insufficient flow:**<br>Desired PIP not reached with mandatory breaths<br>↑ WOB (retractions, etc.)<br>Pressure fluctuations on manometer around baseline PEEP setting<br>Ventilator asynchrony<br>Graphics: displays a characteristic "figure eight" (as patient's demand outstrips delivered flow pressure decreases while volume increases) |

| Flow Waveform | |
|---|---|
| **Clinical Notes** | Decelerating waveforms are generally preferred.<br>See page 11-6 for discussion of waveforms |

| Inspiratory:Expiratory Ratio (I:E Ratio) | |
|---|---|
| Normal Range | 1:1 to 1:3 |
| Clinical Notes | I:E Ratio is usually not set directly. Setting the RR and TI (or Flow Rate) determines the I:E Ratio.<br>$PaCO_2$ is seldom altered significantly by altering I:E Ratio. Altering PIP and PEEP is usually more effective. |
| Cautions | Inverse ratios carry a high risk of auto-PEEP and the potential for hyperinflation, barotrauma, ↓ CO, and cerebral injury |

| Expiratory Time (TE) | |
|---|---|
| Clinical Notes | **TE is usually not set**, but is the result of the rate and TI<br>$TE = (60/f) - TI$ |
| Cautions | Care should be taken to observe expiratory time, which can best be assessed by observing the flow volume loop or scalar, ensuring that exhalation returns to baseline before the next breath begins |

| Oxygen Percentage ($O_2$ %)<br>Fraction of Inspired Oxygen ($FIO_2$) -- decimal equivalent | |
|---|---|
| Normal Range | 0.21 - 1.0<br>(maintain < 0.50 whenever possible) |
| Clinical Notes | Clinical consequences of moderate-to-high levels of oxygen are well documented (free radicals, ↑ inflammatory response, cell damage, etc.). The goal of care is to use the lowest amount of $O_2$ possible to meet minimum oxygenation goals. |

## ■ Noninvasive Positive Pressure Ventilation

**Indications**

Note that this list is flexible. Many clinicians will trial NPPV for various situations, unless contraindicated. However, in pediatric populations there may be challenges with compliance and proper fit of approved interfaces (resulting in a need for intubation).

### Interfaces

Because there is a wide range of ages being treated with NPPV, the appropriate options vary from Nasal CPAP (young infants) to mask BiPAP (adolescents).

| Type of Support | Selection Criteria |
|---|---|
| Nasal CPAP/BiPAP | Preferred method for obligate nose-breathers See N-CPAP in Neonatal Ventilation Chapter |
| Mask CPAP/BiPAP | As children age and the anatomy changes, mask BiPAP becomes appropriate |

*For Physiologic Effects: See Neonatal Ventilation*
*(page 4-22)*

*For Other Interfaces: See Neonatal Ventilation*
*(page 4-23)*

*For N-IMV, SiPAP, N-HFV: See Neonatal Ventilation*
*(page 4-32 to 4-34)*

## Management of Patient on NPPV

| Therapy Phase | Management |
|---|---|
| *Initiating* | • Spending adequate time with the patient may play a major role in compliance<br>• Explain therapy to patient and family<br>• Begin at low settings (EPAP 4-5 cmH$_2$O, IPAP 6-10 cmH$_2$O)<br>• Place mask gently on patient's face, perhaps allow patient (or family) to hold mask on their own face<br>• Do not strap mask on until patient comfortable with pressure<br>• Increase settings as needed and as patient tolerates<br>• Heated humidity is recommended for all patients on NPPV, but is absolutely clinically indicated within several hours following initiation |
| *Managing* | • To increase ventilation (to change pressure support level):<br>    Increase IPAP or<br>    Decrease EPAP<br>• To decrease ventilation (to change pressure support level):<br>    Decrease IPAP or<br>    Increase EPAP<br>• To improve trigger dysynchrony:<br>    *Attempt to increase EPAP (If the same PS is desired, clinician must increase IPAP the same increments as the EPAP)<br>    *If using a critical care ventilator simply change PS level to affect ventilation and change PEEP to address trigger asynchrony |
| *Weaning* | • Begin by decreasing FiO$_2$ and pressure as tolerated<br>• Remove NPPV from patient for short breaks. Monitor for respiratory distress and the need to restart therapy<br>• Breaks may be lengthened to wean further |

## Monitoring for Success

- Once NPPV is initiated, close observation is required to assess efficacy.
- Rapid improvement should occur (1-2 hours) by the following signs:
- *Patient comfort:* ↓ RR, ↓ use of accessory muscles, ↓ dyspnea, synchronization with NPPV.
- *Improvement in $PaCO_2$ / respiratory acidosis*

---

*Criteria for stopping NPPV attempts and initiating alternative therapy (ET intubation):*
- barotrauma
- failure of indications to improve
- hemodynamic instability
- hypercapnia
- inability to accept any of the interfaces attempted
- inability to clear secretions
- pulmonary emboli
- sepsis
- worsening agitation
- worsening mental status
- worsening oxygenation.

---

*Clinical effectiveness is assessed by:*
- Improved oximetry
- Improved clinical assessment
- An elevated $PaCO_2$ does not have to drop; however progressive hypercapnia with the application of NPPV indicates failure.

## ■ CPAP: Initiation and Management

The following are general guidelines.

**Initiate** CPAP at 4-6 cmH$_2$O

       Initiate early for best potential results

**Adjust** CPAP for continued hypoxemia (PaO$_2$ < 50 mm Hg):

1. Increase CPAP by 2 cmH$_2$O, to a total CPAP of 10-12 cmH$_2$O. The goal is to keep O$_2$ < 30-40%.
2. Increase O$_2$ in increments of 5-10% up to 100%
3. Consider intubating (give CPAP via ET Tube)
4. Consider Pressure Support with Volume, or Volume A/C (allow variable pressure and flow)
5. Full support ventilation if determined to be failing CPAP

### Monitoring Patients on CPAP

- Abdominal distension and bowel sounds
- Skin color and integrity
- ABGs or CBGs with SpO$_2$ and ETCO$_2$
- Chest X-Ray (CXR)
- Vital Signs (HR, RR, BP, temperature)
- WOB (RR, pattern, retractions)
- Ensure proper interface - a tight seal is not usually needed
- Proper Sizing:  Nasal prongs should fill nares, but not cause any blanching (which will lead to skin/tissue breakdown)
- CPAP: pressure, pop-off, leaks
- Gas temperature, humidity

### Complications

| | |
|---|---|
| Air leaks | Pulmonary edema |
| Aspiration | Renal dysfunction |
| Feeding intolerance | Respiratory failure |
| Gastric distention/rupture | Sepsis |
| Hypothermia | Tube/prong obstruction, |
| Increased ICP (IVH) | dislodgement, irritation, |
| Infection (if ET Tube) | Nasal necrosis |
| Muscle fatigue | Under- or over-hydration |
| Pneumothorax/PIE | Under- or over-temperature |

## Indications of CPAP Success (and suggested actions)

| Inadequate CPAP (↓)  *Increase CPAP in incrememnts* | Continued respiratory distress  SpO₂ may not change; may gradually worsen  RR: no change or worsens  CXR: no change or worsens |
|---|---|
| **Adequate CPAP** | ↑ PaO₂ (SpO₂)  RR towards normal  ↓ WOB  CXR: improved aeration |
| **Optimal CPAP** | To determine:  1. Look for highest SpO₂ without a significant change in pH/PaCO₂ or CV status  -OR-  2. Point of initial rise in esophageal pressure (3-6 cmH₂O) |
| **Excessive CPAP (↑)**  *Decrease CPAP immediately* | Gastric distention  Vomiting  ↓ Cardiac Output (CV instability)  ↑ PaCO₂, ↓ PaO₂  ↑ Work of breathing |

### Indications of CPAP Failure (any one of the following):
- PaO₂ < 50 mm Hg on 100% O₂, CPAP 10-12 cmH₂O
- Hypercapnia
- pH < 7.20 (respiratory)
- Apnea and bradycardia
- Change in LOC (lethargy, unresponsiveness)
- Respiratory distress

### Selected Causes of CPAP Failure:
- Airway obstruction (pharynx, secretions)
- Apnea
- Atelectasis persisting (ineffective CPAP)
- Insufficient pressure or flow
- Intraventricular hemorrhage (IVH)
- Muscle fatigue (nutrition, prematurity)
- Metabolic acidosis
- Pulmonary edema

## ■ CPAP:

**When to Wean:**
- ABGs improving ($SpO_2 \geq 90\%$ or $PaO_2 \geq 70$ mm Hg) and/or ↓ esophageal pressure
- CXR improving (increased aeration/expansion)
- Any respiratory distress has resolved
- Vital signs stable

**Weaning Process**
1. ↓ $FIO_2$ by 3-5% increments, down to 40%
2. ↓ CPAP by 1 - 2 increments, down to 3 - 4 cm $H_2O$
3. Remove CPAP when $O_2 \leq 40\%$, CPAP 3 - 4 cm $H_2O$, and no respiratory distress for several hours (several days for BPD patients)
4. IF INVASIVE APPLICATION: Extubate ET tube when discontinuing CPAP, due to the high resistance of small ET tubes
5. Place patient on slightly higher $FIO_2$ than was on with CPAP

**Clinical Notes**
- Maintain $SpO_2 \geq 90\%$, $PaO_2$ 50 - 70 mm Hg, $PaCO_2 < 55$ mm Hg, and pH > 7.25
- Move to next step as $SpO_2 > 90\%$ or $PaO_2 > 70$ mm Hg.
- Incremental changes may be made as often as every 2 hours
- Obtain CXR to assess for adequate lung inflation
- Stop wean if $PaO_2 < 50$ mm Hg or retractions increase

# ■ Invasive Ventilation

### Indications for Mechanical Ventilation

- <u>Apnea</u>: prolonged or repetitive, unresponsive apnea associated with bradycardia and/or cyanosis
- <u>Respiratory failure</u>:
  - $PaO_2 < 50$ mm Hg on $FIO_2 \geq 60\%$
  - $PaCO_2 > 60\text{-}65$ mm Hg ( $> 55$ mm Hg in infants $< 1500$ g)
  - pH $< 7.20$
- <u>Impending respiratory failure</u>. While somewhat subjective, the following should be considered:
  - Worsening oxygenation
  - Respiratory distress ($\uparrow$ RR $> 60$ breaths/min; retractions, grunting, nasal flaring)
  - ABG values may or may not be within acceptable ranges

### Contraindications for Mechanical Ventilation
- Lack of consent (relative contraindication)

# ■ Conventional Ventilation: Modes
**Pressure vs. Volume Ventilation**

> There is a general lack of data in the pediatric population supporting any specific mode. It is more important to monitor.

## Pediatric Modes
*Many of these modes have been covered in the Neonatal Ventilation Chapter - reference pages are provided.*

| Pressure Ventilation | Volume Ventilation |
|---|---|
| P-SIMV (SEE page 4-36) | V-SIMV (A) |
| PC-A/C (SEE page 4-38) | VC-A/C (B) |
| PS (SEE page 4-40) | *Volume-targeted modes of ventilation are pressure ventilation (the pressure varies to target a set tidal volume)* |
| **Volume-Targeted Modes** | |
| PRVC (SEE page 4-42) | |
| APV (SEE PRVC) | |
| VG (SEE page 4-44) | |
| **Other** | |
| APRV (C)<br>NAVA (SEE page 4-55)<br>ECMO (D) | *APRV is classified as a pressure mode of ventilation, but due to its unique characteristics it is included in this category* |
| **High Frequency** | |
| HFOV (SEE page 4-67) | HFJV (SEE page 4-75) |

# Volume - Synchronized Intermittent Mandatory Ventilation   **A**
(V-SIMV or V/C-SIMV)

| Summary | A combination of spontaneous and mandatory ventilation. |
|---|---|
| | • The ventilator will deliver a set number of mandatory (controlled) breaths per minute. |
| | • These mandatory breaths will be at a preset $V_T$ and $\dot{V}_I$ |
| | • The patient may breathe spontaneously in between the mandatory machine breaths from the baseline pressure. The breath may be assisted with pressure support. |
| | • If the patient begins to inspire just prior to the time-triggered mandatory (control) breath, a full machine-assisted breath will be delivered. |
| | Pressure-supported breaths may ↑ patient comfort, while controlled breaths (with longer TI) ensure mPAW and lung recruitment |

| | Classified By: | | |
|---|---|---|---|
| **Breath Type** | **Trigger** | **Limit** | **Cycle** |
| **Mandatory** *(Controlled)* | MT *(Time)* | ML *($\dot{V}$ or Vol)* | MC *(Vol)* |
| **Assisted** | PT *(Press or $\dot{V}$)* | ML *($\dot{V}$ or Vol)* | MC *(Vol)* |
| **Spontaneous** | PT *(Press or $\dot{V}$)* | PL *(Press)* | PC *(Press or $\dot{V}$)* |

MT = Machine-triggered    PT = Patient-triggered
ML = Machine-limited      PL = Patient-limited
MC = Machine-cycled      PC = Patient-cycled

**Indications:**
• Full to partial ventilatory support

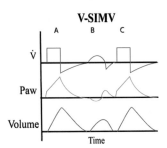

**V-SIMV**

Breath A is Controlled + Time triggered
Breath B is a spontaneous breath (no pressure support)
Breath C is synchronized and assisted
Breaths A + C are both full machine volume breaths

**Advantages:**
- More tightly controls volume with each mandatory breath.
- Security of a safe minimum $\dot{V}_E$
- May maintain respiratory muscle strength (avoids atrophy)
- Synchronization of spontaneous and mandatory breaths
- Spontaneous breaths may be pressure supported (see PSV)
- Spontaneous breathing generally produces better gas distribution and less cardiac output compromise

**Disadvantages and Risks:**
- High pressure limit must be set appropriately to minimize the risk of alveolar injury
- Patient work of breathing increased if flow rate/sensitivity are not set correctly
- Possible tachypnea with fatigue and hypercapnia if mandatory (control) rate is set too low (inadequate ventilatory support or weaning too rapidly)
- ↑ patient work of breathing for spontaneous breaths unless adequate PSV is added

# Volume Control / Assist-Control
(VC/AC or V-A/C or V/C-A/C)

| Summary | • A combination of assisted and/or controlled (mandatory) ventilation.<br>• All breaths are delivered at a set $V_T$ and $\dot{V}_I$<br>• In between the controlled (set rate) breaths, a patient can trigger a full machine (assisted) breath at the same parameters as the controlled breath (i.e., $V_T$ and $\dot{V}_I$). |
|---|---|

### Other Names for Volume-Assist/Control

Volume Control
Volume Assist Mechanical Ventilation
Continuous Mechanical Ventilation (CMV)
Assist/Control Volume Control (AC/VC)

| Other Names for Assist | Other Names for Control |
|---|---|
| Assisted Ventilation (AV) | Control Mode |
| Assisted Mechanical Ventilation (AMV) | Controlled Mechanical Ventilation (CMV) |
| Volume Assist (VA) | Controlled Mandatory Ventilation (CMV) |
| Volume Cycled Ventilation (VCV) | Volume Control Ventilation (VCV) |
| | Volume Cycled Ventilation (VCV) |

| | Classified By: | | |
|---|---|---|---|
| Breath Type | Trigger | Limit | Cycle |
| **Mandatory** *(Controlled)* | MT *(Time)* | ML *($\dot{V}$ or Vol)* | MC *(Vol)* |
| **Assisted** | PT *(Press or $\dot{V}$)* | ML *($\dot{V}$ or Vol)* | MC *(Vol)* |

MT = Machine-triggered  PT = Patient-triggered
ML = Machine-limited  PL = Patient-limited
MC = Machine-cycled  PC = Patient-cycled

**Indications**:

• Patients requiring full ventilatory support. For those who make inadequate or no respiratory effort due to: drugs, cerebral malfunction, spinal cord or phrenic nerve injury, or motor nerve paralysis.
• Used in patients with stable respiratory drives who are able to trigger the ventilator.

## V-ACV

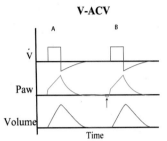

Breath A is Controlled + Machine-Triggered
Breath B is Assisted + Patient-Triggered
Each Breath is a Full Machine-Pressure Breath

**Advantages**:
- Maximum ventilatory support
- Guaranteed $V_T$ with a minimum $\dot{V}_E$
- Minimal patient WOB (if parameters are properly adjusted)
- Allows some patient control of $f$ and $\dot{V}_E$

**Disadvantages**:
- High pressure limit must be set appropriately to minimize the risk of alveolar injury
- The flow is fixed, which inhibits the patient who has a ↑ $\dot{V}_I$ or volume demand.
- High risk of cardiovascular compromise
- May be poorly tolerated in awake, nonsedated patients
- May cause or worsen auto-PEEP (dynamic hyperinflation)

# ▓ Conventional Ventilation: Management

### Initiating Invasive Ventilation
*See Parameters for guidelines on initiating ventilation*

*There are no rules or definitive guidelines for ventilation, only sugges-
tions. All settings are variable and must be modified based upon the
disease state, ventilation type, gestational age, postnatal age, and
weight.*

*The goal should be to carefully support oxygen and ventilation needs
while avoiding complications, particularly any harm.*

### Summary Overview of Initial Settings:

| Parameter | Pediatric Setting |
|---|---|
| (Mode) | no specific mode is supported by evidence |
| $V_T$ | ~ 6 mL/kg IBW |
| PIP (Inspiratory Pressure) | 15-20 cm $H_2O$  ( < 30 cm $H_2O$) |
| PEEP | 4-7 cm $H_2O$ |
| $T_I$ | Varies by age of child |
| $FIO_2$ | As minimal as possible to maintain $SpO_2$ goal range |

> **See Specific Diseases/Disorders in Chapter 10
> for specific recommendations, when available.**

## Oxygenation

In general, oxygenation goals are very conservative.

| Improving Oxygenation: $PaO_2$ ($SaO_2$, $SpO_2$) | |
|---|---|
| Goal | To maintain adequate $O_2$ delivery to the tissues while ventilating with the lowest possible $FiO_2$ and pressures. |
| | **Permissive (severe pediatric ARDS):** Maintain SpO₂ as low as 85-92% *(assumes stable hemodynamic status)* |
| Methods: Details | ↑ FiO₂: Immediate but temporary measure for increasing the $O_2$ gradient |
| See following pages | Optimize mPAW: $V_T$, PIP, PEEP, $T_I$, $\dot{V}I$, $\dot{V}I$ waveform. This has a greater effect on V/Q matching and is often a key to improving and support oxygenation. |
| | Adequate $O_2$ delivery to tissues is dependent on $FiO_2$, CO, and $CaO_2$. |

## Quick Estimates of Oxygenation Status:

**P/F ratio** = $PaO_2 / F_iO_2$
- $PaO_2$ is the amount of oxygen in the arteries
- $FIO_2$ is the amount of oxygen in the alveoli (roughly, of course)
- The ratio estimates how well oxygen is getting from alveoli to the arteries.
- Normal is approximately 500

**Oxygen Index (OI)** = $\dfrac{F_iO_2 \times Paw \times 100}{PaO_2}$ $\qquad$ $F_iO_2$ is a decimal!

OI also estimates the amount of oxygen that goes from alveoli to blood, but takes into account mean airway pressure, which we know is greatly impacted by factors like PEEP. Thus, the OI can be considered a more powerful estimate of oxygenation.

## Methods for Improving Oxygenation
*see details on following pages*

Concept: Increasing FIO₂ is a temporary measure, but has severe consequences for neonates. Optimizing mPAW is critical.

1. Increase $FIO_2$ (↑ $O_2$ tension/gradient)
2. Optimize mPAW by PEEP
   (eliminate auto-PEEP, ↑ FRC, ↓ shunting)
3. Optimize mPAW other than by PEEP (↑ FRC)
4. Position Patient (optimize V/Q matching)

| 1. F₁O₂ | |
|---------|---|
| **Goal** | Use the minimum amount of supplemental oxygen necessary to maintain <u>adequate</u> oxygenation (not necessarily normal oxygenation) |
| **Principle** | This is a major determinant of oxygenation, increasing the $P(A\text{-}a)O_2$ gradient, which usually results in a greater $PaO_2$. |
| **Clinical Notes** | Increase $F_IO_2$ cautiously. High $F_IO_2$ over time may lead to Oxygen Toxicity, so the overall goal is to maintain as low clinically possible. It is often preferred to optimize mPAW versus chasing the patient's SpO₂ using $F_IO_2$. |

| 2. PEEP | |
|---|---|
| Goal | OPTIMAL PEEP which: <br> ↑ PaO$_2$ – ↓ shunt effect, ↑ FRC, and ↑ CL, allowing for the reduction of FiO$_2$ and its complications. <br> ↓ **WOB** – Unload the inspiratory muscles (esp. in diseases like BPD). |
| Principle | Determinant of oxygenation by affecting Paw. |
| Clinical Notes | Maintains pressures above ambient pressure during the expiratory phase to prevent collapse of smaller airways and unstable alveoli. |
| Contraindications | **Absolute:** <br> Tension or untreated pneumothorax <br><br> **Relative:** <br><br> • Barotrauma <br> • Bronchopulmonary fistula <br> • Pre-existing hyperinflation <br><br> • Hypovolemia <br> • Recent lung surgery <br> • Unilateral lung disorders |

**Beneficial Effects of Appropriate PEEP**

↑ $\overline{Paw}$    ↑ CL    ↑ PaO$_2$ (for a given FiO$_2$)    ↓ WOB

↑ V/Q (the stabilization of collapsing alveoli resulting in improved gas distribution and ↓ R-L shunting).

↑ FRC (which may include recruitment of collapsed alveoli)

↓ Lung injury (minimizes shear forces)

PEEP may be beneficial in patients with CHF by ↓ preload and afterload.

**Potential Adverse Effects of PEEP**

Alveolar over-distension (volutrauma, which is proportional to lung disease, over-distension, and pressure), ↑ WOB, ↑ V$_D$/V$_T$.

CV Effects are dependent on PEEP level, C$_{LT}$, and CV status. The greatest effect (↓ venous return and CO) is when lung compliance is high, chest wall compliance is low, and cardiovascular reserve is low.

May ↓ renal and portal blood flow, which results in ↓ urinary output.

When PEEP decreases venous return, ICP may ↑. This is usually clinically insignificant unless ICP is already elevated. Elevating the head may offset PEEP effect on ICP.

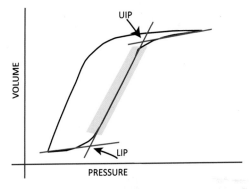

## Understanding the P-V Loop and PEEP:

1. The steep part of the curve represents rapid increases in Volume with small pressure changes, implying best compliance as the lungs accept volume easily.

2. The flattened sections represent areas where it takes greater pressures to move small volumes of air (the cost of ventilation, and the risk of lung damage, is high):

   **Lower**: Lower flattened section suggests areas of the lungs that are closing and opening, which results in atelectrauma. These are separated in the above diagram by the Lower Inflection Point (LIP).

   **Upper**: Upper flattened section ("duckbill"), when present, suggests over-distension, which can lead to barotrauma (damage caused by excessive pressure). PEEP should always be set below the Upper Inflection Point (UIP).

3. The slope of the curve provides information about lung compliance. Less steep curves suggest poor compliance (it always takes a fair amount of pressure to deliver a volume)

4. Ideally this curve is captured with no patient contribution, meaning it is most accurate when a patient is given a single-dose of a paralytic. Note that the LIP in particular is not always discernible.

| 3. Mean Airway Pressure ($\overline{Paw}$ or MAWP or MAP or mPAW) | |
|---|---|
| Goal | Achieve adequate oxygenation with the lowest possible pressures and $F_IO_2$ without impairing CV function or injury to the lungs |
| Principle | Paw is an important determinant of oxygenation<br><br>$PaO_2 \sim \overline{Paw}$<br>     (until over-distension occurs - see pg 11-31) |
| Indication | ↑ Paw is indicated for patients with ↓ lung volumes and refractory hypoxemia (does not respond to increasing the $F_IO_2$)<br><br>Refractory Hypoxemia =<br>     $PaO_2 < 60$ mmHg on $F_IO_2 > 0.6$ |

**Primary Factors Affecting $\overline{Paw}$** (in probable order of influence)

- PEEP
- PIP
- $T_I$
- $f$ (↓ $T_E$)
- $\dot{V}_I$
- $\dot{V}_I$ waveform

Clinical Note: Limit $T_I$ to the maximum that does not cause auto-PEEP.
If auto-PEEP present:   In VV: auto-PEEP → ↑Palv ($V_T$ constant)
                      In PV: auto-PEEP → ↓ $V_T$ (Palv constant)

**Potential Risks of** ↑ $\overline{Paw}$ = barotrauma, ↓ CO

**Measurement Of $\overline{Paw}$**

| Automatically calculated by ventilator | Manually calculated |
|---|---|
| Note: this value usually doesn't include any auto-PEEP | $\overline{Paw} = (PIP - PEEP) \times (T_I / T_{total}) + PEEP$ (figuring a constant flow, VV breath and PEEP includes auto-PEEP) |

Pediatric

Ventilation

| 4. Patient Positioning | |
|---|---|
| **Goal** | Improve V/Q and FRC by placing patient in various positions — usually either lateral (right side down or left side down) or by proning patient (stomach down) |
| **Principle** | This may assist with oxygenation by aligning perfusion (blood will go wherever gravity takes it down) WITH ventilation (placing the better lung regions where the best perfusion is). You are aligning good lung with good perfusion, as much as possible.<br><br>BLU GLD (remember it as: Blue Gold) =<br>               Bad Lung UP, Good Lung DOWN<br>(Except with pulmon. hemorrhage, lung abscess) |
| **Contrain-dication** | **Absolute**:<br>Spinal cord instability<br>**Relative**:<br>Thoracic/abdominal surgeries (recent)<br>Hemodynamic/cardiovascular instability |
| **Clinical Notes** | • Careful monitoring of ventilator parameters and patient deterioration, complications, line/tube placement, etc., is essential during and directly following repositioning<br>• Improvement is most likely within 30 minutes |

**Procedure**:
- Ensure team members are in place (including 1 person in charge of monitoring secure airway/vent circuit)
- Unhook all leads/lines as necessary
- Gently place patient on side
- Verify status of patient/equipment/lines
- Place patient in prone position
- Turn patient's head towards the ventilator
- Reattach and verify all leads/lines - ensure that the ET tube/head are not compressed
- Do a complete ventilator-patient check, including breath sounds
- Again verify vital signs and hemodynamic status

## Ventilation

| | Improving Ventilation: PaCO$_2$ (and pH) |
|---|---|
| **Goal** | Maintain adequate CO$_2$ elimination while protecting the lungs from injury. |
| **Principle** | Adequacy of ventilation is mostly determined by minute ventilation, and assessed by PaCO$_2$/pH (Several therapeutic strategies exist, including lung protection) |
| | PaCO$_2$ and resultant pH are impacted by total ventilation, deadspace, and CO$_2$ production. They are changed by altering minute ventilation, deadspace and/or CO$_2$ production. Note that deadspace is not often used therapeutically anymore. |
| **Methods** | **Manipulating ventilation occurs in two ways:** |
| | 1. **Tidal Volume** ($\Delta$P in pressure control modes) Typically set to a range based upon height (ideal body weight). There is usually wiggle room within that range for minor adjustments, but ultimately is a "set and forget" parameter. |
| | 2. **Ventilator Rate ($f$)** More typically manipulated to alter minute ventilation in either volume or pressure control modes. Changing $f$ also changes I:E ratio, so care must be taken to ensure adequate exhalation time. |
| | Manipulating these parameters is dependent on mode, patient's spontaneous (total) rate, spontaneous tidal volume in some modes, inspiratory time, disease process, etc. |
| | **Independent of disease processes:** <br> • $\uparrow$ VT, $\Delta$P, or RR will $\uparrow$ Minute Ventilation, which therefore $\downarrow$ CO$_2$ and $\uparrow$ pH <br> • $\downarrow$ VT, $\Delta$P, or RR will $\downarrow$ Minute Ventilation, which therefore $\uparrow$ CO$_2$ and $\downarrow$ pH |

# Additonal Methods of Improving Ventilation

## Respiratory Acidosis
- Allow for permissive hypercapnia
  (allow $CO_2$ to rise and pH to fall to a minimal safe level)
- Increase spontaneous tidal volume
  - Pressure support
  - Short-acting beta agonist
  - Increase ET Tube size
  - Nutritional consult
- Decrease mechanical deadspace
  - Use low compliance circuit
  - Cut ET tube shorter
  - Consider tracheotomy
- High frequency ventilation
- Patient positioning (improves V/Q)
- Verify adequate I:E ratio (flow waveform)
- $\downarrow CO_2$ production: consider fever, surgeries, trauma, sepsis

## Respiratory Alkalosis
- Try pressure support or SIMV
- Sedation (extreme agitation, fear, pain, $\uparrow$ WOB)
- Add mechanical deadspace (not often used clinically)

**If patient is hyperventilating due to hypoxemia
correct the hypoxemia first**

**Tachypnea is often caused by a metabolic acidosis,
so be aware of ABG**

# ■ Conventional Ventilation: Weaning

- Signs that suggest weaning/discontinuation should be initiated:
  - Stable respiratory status (4-8 hours), as evidenced by blood gases, improved P/V loops, etc.
    Adequate spontaneous $\dot{V}_E$
  - Improvement in CXR
  - Stable hemodynamic status (vasopressors, etc.)
- Parameters should be changed frequently and gradually (not slowly with large decreases).
- Careful monitoring should occur during the weaning phase

**Oxygenation:**
- Decrease $FIO_2$ first, then
- Decrease PEEP if > physiologic
  (don't drop below 4-5 cm $H_2O$)

**Ventilation**
- If Pressure Mode: Decrease PIP until < 12 cm $H_2O$
- If Volume Targeted Mode: Decrease target tidal volume
- If in SIMV, consider ↓ $f$ (see SIMV for notes)

**Extubation**
- There are no definitive guidelines. The decision is somewhat subjective.
- Stop feeding 4 hrs before extubation
- Consider extubating to noninvasive positive pressure ventilation (NPPV). SEE Noninvasive Ventilation page 11-15
- Stridor: Consider administering Racemic epinephrine

## Airway Pressure Release Ventilation
(APRV)

| Summary | Primarily a spontaneous mode of ventilation (spontaneous breaths deliver maximum therapeutic advantage). This mode is basically "inverse ratio" ventilation if patient is not breathing spontaneously. |
|---|---|

Patient is able to breathe at two pressure levels:

1. A longer high level which allows for alveolar recruitment -- This is referred to as Phigh (the set pressure) and Thigh (the set time) in traditional form
2. A very short low level (set to therapeutically cause air trapping) -- This is referred to as Plow (the set pressure) and Tlow (the set time) in traditional form
   The purpose of the low level, also called "the release" is to allow for $CO_2$ elimination, while maintaining therapeutic air-trapping.

While controversial, Pressure Support may be added for the spontaneous component of the breath either at high level (all forms of the mode) and sometimes at the low level (Bi-Vent)

**Other Names:** Bilevel, BiPAP[1], CPAP with release, Intermittent CPAP, Variable Positive Airway Pressure (VPAP)

|  | Classified By: | | |
|---|---|---|---|
| **Breath Type** | **Trigger** | **Limit** | **Cycle** |
| **Mandatory** *(Controlled)* | MT *(Time)* | ML *(Pressure)* | MC *(Vol)* |
| **Assisted** | PT *(Press or Flow)* | ML *(Pressure)* | MC *(Press or Flow)* |

[1] **Name Alert!** This is not the same BiPAP term used in noninvasive ventilation.

## APRV Initial Suggested Settings

| | |
|---|---|
| **P high** (high pressure level) | 15-30 cm $H_2O$<br>The lower the patient's P/F ratio (or higher the OI), the higher the initial setting needed |
| **T high** (time spent at high pressure level) | 4-6 seconds<br>T high should be 80-95% of the total cycle time. This provides a relatively high mPAW, preventing collapse of unstable alveoli and recruiting additional alveolar units |
| **P low** (low pressure level) | 0 cm $H_2O$<br>Allows for maximum ΔP for unimpeded expiratory flow. Setting above zero may add expiratory resistance, inhibiting $CO_2$ removal |
| **T low** (time spent at low pressure level) | The actual value is less important than using waveform interpretation—graphics (typically initial setting is 0.4-0.6 seconds).<br><br>Use flow scalar or loop to set expiratory flow termination point to 50-75% of peak expiratory flow. In essense it is creating intentional auto-PEEP (not allowing flow to return to baseline during exhalation) |
| **Trigger** | Set to avoid auto-triggering; may require pressure trigger |
| **Pressure Support** | Use of any pressure support is debated. While it may decrease work of breathing, it can also lead to higher transpulmonary pressures (including ↑ risk of overdistension which would offset any gains in V/Q matching) |

**There is limited data to support or contradict the use of APRV with infants and children.**

## APRV Management

Since spontaneous ventilation is an integral part of APRV, a change in the vent settings may not elicit as great a change in $PaCO_2$ as would occur with conventional MV.

- Maintaining the lungs as "open" (P high and T high do this - in essence doing a recruitment maneuver) improves V/Q and may recruit collapsed alveolar units
- Spontaneous ventilation (primarily during T high)
- Release time (T low)—these releases "dump" CO2
- During prolonged T high, cardiac output continuously delivers $CO_2$ from the bood into the alveolar space. As the airways remain open, cardiogenic mixing results in $CO_2$ movement into the central airways, with reduced anatomical deadspace.
- Attempts to use the machine in a conventional method (decreasing the T high and increasing T low in an attempt to increase the "cycling" or "dumps") may actually have the opposite effect (a reduction in $CO_2$ elimination and oxygenation).

### Improving Oxygenation on APRV (Goal: ↑ $PaO_2$)

| | |
|---|---|
| **P high** (high pressure level) | **Increase** in 2-5 cm H2O increments (up to 30, maybe 40 with low compliance). Monitor hemodynamic status. |
| **T high** (time spent at high pressure level) | **Increase** by 0.5-2 sec, along with P high increases (may go up to 10-15 seconds) |
| **T low** (time spent at low pressure level) | **Decrease** T low in 0.1 sec increments towards expiratory flow termination of 75% of PEF (increases end expiratory lung volume). Caution: May decrease VT, which will ↑ CO2 |
| **FIO₂** | Keep FiO₂ as low as clinically indicated |
| **Recruitment** | Consider recruitment maneuvers if ncessary (e.g. Phigh 40-50 and Thigh 30-60) |

## Improving Ventilation on APRV (Goal: ↓ PaCO₂)

| P high (high pressure level) | **Increase** in 2-5 cm H₂O increments (up to 30, maybe 40 with low compliance). Increases ΔP, increasing expiratory flow and CO₂ elimination. Monitor tidal volume hemodynamic status. |
|---|---|
| T high (time spent at high pressure level) | **Preferred Method:** **Increase** T high in 0.5-0.1 increments, along with P high increases (may go up to 10-15 seconds). Monitor VT/hemo status. It increases minute ventilation by increasing ΔP, while preserving FRC (the T high, in part, does this) **Less Preferred Method (do preferred first!):** **Decrease** T high in 0.5-0.1 increments simultaneously with increasing Phigh. This increases minute ventilation by allowing for more releases, but may decrease mPAW (affecting oxygenation). |
| T low (time spent at low pressure level) | **Increase** Tlow in 0.5-0.1 increments towards 50% PEF to allow more time for exhalation. This may lead to airway closure/derecruitment (oxygenation status should be acceptable) |
| Titrate sedation | Target RASS score -2 to 0 |
| Maintain pH | Hypercapnia may be required to maintain pH > 7.25 |

## Improving Ventilation on APRV (Goal: ↑ PaCO₂)

| P high (high pressure level) | **Decrease** in 2-5 cm H₂O increments if oxygenation status is acceptable. This decreases ΔP, decreasing expiratory flow and CO₂ elimation. |
|---|---|
| T high (time spent at high pressure level) | **Increase** slowly in increments of 0.5-2 seconds. This reduces number of releases. |

## Weaning APRV

1. **Wean FiO₂ first.** Target is < 50%
2. **"Drop and Stretch"** (Habashi method).
   Do these simultaneously:

| | |
|---|---|
| **DROP**<br>**P high**<br>(high pressure level)<br><br>**AND** | **Decrease** in 2-5 cm H₂O increments ONLY after FiO₂ < 50% and oxygenation status stable for 2 hours.<br><br>Continue until 16-20 cmH₂O (maintaining desired PaCO₂)<br><br>This all results in lower mPAW |
| **STRETCH**<br>**T high**<br>(time spent at high pressure level) | **Increase** T high in 0.5 increments up to 15 seconds. This decreases the number of releases and allows for a greater time for spontaneous ventiation during T high.<br><br>At 15 seconds, the release rate is only 4/min - minimal. |

3. **Reach CPAP**
   Note that some clinicians transition to a conventional mode of ventilation, such as PSV at this time.
   - The goal is to progress towards pure CPAP, by decreasing P high and increasing T high (Drop and Stretch).
   - The child's spontaneous rate should be increasing to compensate
   - When P high is around 16 with T high of 12-15 seconds, switch to CPAP
   - Titrate CPAP down
   - Consider extubation when CPAP 5-10 cm H₂O

## Extracorporeal Membrane Oxygenation D
(ECMO, ECCO₂R))

| Summary | Blood is circulated out of the body (through cannulization), where it is run through artificial membranes (diffusion, hollow-fiber), allowing for molecular oxygen and carbon dioxide diffusion. The blood then re-enters the body through another cannula. |
|---|---|
| Goal | Allow time for the intrinsic recovery of the lungs and/or heart, or provide the means to medically maintain the patient until organ transplantation is possible. The amount of rest the systems receive is dependent in part on the type of support being provided (see next page). |
| Techniques | • Extracorporeal Membrane Oxygenation (ECMO)<br>• Extracorporeal Carbon Dioxide Removal (ECCO₂R) |

# Types of Support

**Venoarterial (VA)** *provides heart and lung support:*

| Deoxygenated Blood | actively pumped through oxygenator | Oxygenated Blood |
|---|---|---|
| **Venous Blood** | | **Arterial Blood Supply** |
| Right Atrium | $O_2$ diffuses in $CO_2$ diffuses out | Ascending aorta (Central ECMO) |
| Internal Jugular Vein | | Internal Carotid Artery |

- Decreases cardiac work
- Decreases cardiac oxygen consumption
- Proportion of blood flow can continue through lungs

**Venovenous (VV)** *provides lung support:*

| Deoxygenated Blood | actively pumped through oxygenator | Oxygenated Blood |
|---|---|---|
| **Venous Blood** | | **Venous Blood Supply** |
| Single Dual-Lumen Cannula in the Internal Jugular Vein | | Single Dual-Lumen Cannula in the Internal Jugular Vein |
| Blood enters the cannula through the lower port (usually in Inferior Vena Cava) | $O_2$ diffuses in $CO_2$ diffuses out | Blood exits the cannula through the proximal port (usually in the right atrium) |

- Does not support circulation
- May recirculate previously oxygenated blood (depends on cannula placement)
- $ECCO_2R$ allows for oxygenation by lungs, $CO_2$ removal by ECMO
- Femoral access is not indicated in children < 10 kg

## Initiation Criteria

*Note that ECMO indications vary and are changing rapidly*

| Neonatal Criteria | |
|---|---|
| Disease criteria | • Asphyxia<br>• Congential diaphragmatic hernia (CDH)<br>• Persistent pulmonary hypertension of the new-born (PPHN)<br>• Meconium aspiration syndrome (MAS)<br>• Respiratory distress syndrome (RDS)<br>• Group B streptococcal sepsis |
| Clinical criteria | • > 34-weeks gestation<br>• Birth weight ≥ 2 kg<br>• No coagulopathy (or bleeding)<br>• No major intracranial hemorrhage (Grade 1)<br>• Mechanical Ventilation < 14 days<br>  • A-a gradient (600-624 mm Hg for 4-12 hrs)<br>  • Oxygen Index (> 40 for > 4 hours)<br>   (or OI > 20 with lack of improvement despite maximized supports)<br>  • Progressive respiratory failure and/or pulmonary hypertension<br>   (RV dysfunction, ↑ inotropics)<br>• Reversible lung injury<br>• No untreatable major conditions (cardiac, malformations)<br>• Routine therapies have been maximized |
| **Pediatric Criteria** | |
| Disease criteria | • Status asthmaticus ($CO_2$ removal)<br>• Surgical repair of tracheobronchial tree<br>• Mediastinal mass (causing airway compression)<br>• Pulmonary embolism<br>• Pediatric ARDS (with shock, trauma, sepsis)<br>• Massive fluid overload |
| Clinical criteria | Within 1st 7-days of high levels of mechanical ventilation support |

### Relative Contraindications

- Evidence of ischemic neurological damage
- Structural (congenital) cardiac disease
- Severe hypoxemia (prolonged)
- Mechanical ventilation (prolonged > 7 days)

### Absolute Contraindications

- Weight < 2 kg and/or age < 35 wks gestational
- Severe asphyxia or ischemia
- Poor underlying prognosis (trisomy 13, trisomy 18, etc.)
- Anticoagulation contraindications (numerous)

### Ventilator Management

| Patient / Goal | Typical Settings |
|---|---|
| **Cardiac patients** Goal: maintain lung function near normal | Pressure Assist/Control PIP ~ 25 cm $H_2O$ (VT 5-7 mL/kg IBW) PEEP 5 cm $H_2O$ f: 10-12 breaths/min |
| **Respiratory patients** Goal: allow lungs to rest while preventing atelectasis. | Pressure Assist/Control PIP ~20-25 cm $H_2O$ (VT 4-6 mL/kg IBW) PEEP 4-10 cm $H_2O$ f: 4-10 breaths/min |

- For <u>vent rest</u>: once vent support is set, generally ABGs are managed on the ECMO side (don't fix with the ventilator)
- With VV ECMO SpO₂ will be lower (> 85%)
- Wean ventilator FIO₂ once stabilized on ECMO
- "Whited out" CXR is expected for first 24-hours of support

### ECMO Weaning/discontinuation

- Weaning is the gradual reduction of ECMO *blood flow* and *sweep gas rates* over a period of hours-to-days with simultaneous increase in ventilatory support (as ECMO flow decreases, ventilator settings, including FIO₂, will need to increase as more blood is circulating naturally).
- When flow rates reach 10-30 mL/kg/min, the patient may be isolated from the ECMO circuit
- Alternatively, a trial separation from ECMO support may be performed (with appropriate ventilator support)

# ■ Pediatric Chronic Home Invasive Ventilation[1]

*American Thoracic Society (ATS)*
*Clinical Practice Guideline*

1. Comprehensive medical home co-managed by a generalist and respiratory specialist
2. Readiness for care in the home should be assessed through standardized processes prior to discharge
3. An awake, attentive, trained caregiver should be available at all times
4. A minimum of 2 specifically trained family caregivers should be prepared
5. Ongoing education should occur with the trained family caregivers
6. A pulse oximeter should be used for monitoring in addition to ventilator alarms
7. The following should be available in-home:
   - ventilator
   - back-up ventilator
   - batteries
   - self-inflating bag and mask
   - portable suction equipment
   - heated humidifier
   - supplemental oxygen (for emergency use)
   - small volume nebulizer
   - pulse oximeter
8. If ineffective cough, a Cough Assist device should be available

[1] Summarized from: Sterni LM, Collaco JM, Baker CD, Carroll JL, Sharma GD, Brozek JL, et al. An Official American Thoracic Society CLinical Practice Guideline: Pediatric Chronic Home Invasive Ventilation. American Journal of Respiratory and Critical Care Medicine 2016;193(8):19.

**CONTENTS**

Information presented that is relevant to the American Heart Association's Pediatric Advanced Life Support (PALS) curriculum is noted with this symbol

## Aerosol Delivery Devices

| Type | Use | Comments |
|------|-----|----------|
| **Small Volume Nebulizer (SVN)**<br><br>*Also called handheld, mini-neb, mainstream, sidestream, slipstream, or in-line* | Used to deliver intermittent aerosolized medications<br>Short-term use only<br>Usually 2-5 mL of solution<br>Optimal gas flow rates 6-8 L/min<br>Average particle size 1-5 μm dia | Can be used with a mouthpiece, face mask, trach-collar, T-piece, or ventilator circuit, with normal breathing pattern and with all patients<br>Need electrical, battery, or gas source to power<br>Requires drug preparation<br>Units can be either pneumatic or ultrasonic<br>Use air, not oxygen, for patients on a hypoxic drive.<br>Patient should take periodic deep breaths |
| **Large Volume Nebulizer (LVN) (jet)** | Used for continuous oxygen +/or aerosol therapy (heated or cool).<br>Variable particle size<br>1-2 mL/min output | Can be used with a face mask, trach-collar, or T-piece.<br>Condensation collects in tubing (use a rainout bag)<br>Correct solution level must be maintained<br>↑risk of nosocomial infection<br>Used primarily for patients with tracheostomies. |
| **Ultrasonic (USN) Nebulizer** | Used to mobilize thick secretions in the lower airways<br>90% of particles are 1-5 μm dia<br>Usually only intermittent, but may be continuous therapy.<br>1- 6 mL/min output | Drug preparation required<br>Heat generated by USN may affect bronchodilators<br>May precipitate bronchospasm, overmobilization of secretions, or overhydration.<br>Not all drugs (e.g., Budesonide and Dornase) are compatible with ultrasonic nebulizers.<br>Provides 100% humidity (continuous) |

| Type | Use | Comments |
|------|-----|----------|
| **Metered Dose Inhaler (MDI)** | Intermittent delivery of aerosolized medications.<br><br>Particle size 3-6 μm | First method of choice.  Small, easily cleaned<br>Efficacy is design and technique dependent<br>Inexpensive, convenient, portable, and no drug prep required<br>Inspiratory flow rates should be ≤ 30 LPM<br>May be used in-line with ventilators<br>Patient self-administered, hence may not be appropriate for pediatric or geriatric patients.<br>Requires hand-breath coordination, synchronization with inspiration, and a 4-10 sec. breath hold.<br>Spacer or holding chamber is recommended, esp. with children. |
| **Dry Powder Inhaler (DPI)** | Intermittent delivery of a powdered medication.<br><br>Particle size 1-2 μm | Breath actuated and patient self-administered<br>Breath holding not required<br>High humidity may affect some drugs.<br>Many drugs unavailable in DPI form<br>Not recommended for patients < 6 yrs or with acute broncho-spasm<br>Some units require high flow rates (> 40 Lpm), hence may not be appropriate for pediatric or geriatric patients. |

# Continuous Nebulization

- Several medications can be nebulized continually, though albuterol is most common.
- Dosaging is in mg/hr and can be done a few ways:
  - IV Pump (e.g., AeroGEN)—see manufacturer literature
  - Large volume nebulizers (HOPE or HEART)—see below

**HEART large volume nebulizer**
Gas flow: 10-15 L/min
Aerosol output: 30-50 mL/min

**Take note of varying units of measurement**

**HOPE large volume nebulizer**
Gas flow: 10-15 L/min
Aerosol output: 25 mL/min

## Large volume nebulizer procedure
1. **Determine number of hours nebulizer should run**
   *typically not more than 3-4 hours because dosage can change*

2. **Place desired amount of albuterol (5 mg/mL) in large volume nebulizer cup**

   Amount of albuterol (mL)=
   $$\left(\frac{\text{Desired mg/hr}}{5}\right) \times \text{Desired \# hours}$$

3. **ADD saline up to desired total output**
   *the aerosol output/hr must be known to do this, which is usually secondarily dependent on gas flow to the nebulizer. This is found in the manufacturer's literature.*

   Amount of saline (mL) =
   [(LVN Output (mL/min) x 60) x (Desired # hours)] -
   [albuterol added (mL)]

   **Clinicians will often use preparation charts to minimize error. If calculating, confirm math with another clinician/pharmacy.**

# ◼ Airway Management

Additional detailed airway management information can be found in Oakes' Respiratory Care Pocket Guide (respiratorybooks.com)

## Assessing the Pediatric Airway

1. Be aware of anatomical variations in the Pediatric Airway (SEE page 11-4)
2. Assess the airway

**Mallampati Scoring System**

| I | II | III | IV |
|---|---|---|---|
| | | | |
| Soft palate visible | Soft palate visible | Soft palate visible | Soft palate NOT visible |
| Uvula visible Pillars visible | Uvula visible | Base of uvula visible | Uvula NOT visible |
| Generally uncomplicated airway management | | Potentially difficult airway management (including intubation) | |

## Manual Resuscitation (Bag Valve Mask)

- Self-inflating bags deliver 30%-80 oxygen unless a reservoir bag is attached (then 60-95%). Delivered $O_2$ is affected by Rate, Vt, and peak inspiratory flowrate.
- Pop-off valves are found on many infant/pediatric self-inflating bags. This valve should be closed during CPR or when lung resistance and compliance is poor.
- Some valve designs do not provide continuous flow of $O_2$ to the mask—the bag must be squeezed to open the valve or sufficient inspiratory force created by the child
- PEEP valves should be used in conjunction with the bag-valve-mask when CPAP is indicated (but should not be used in spontaneously-breathing children)
- Positioning: goal is sniffing position (neck flexed forward to the shoulders with head extended). Do not hyperextend as this risks obstructing the airway.

### Effective Ventilation Algorithm

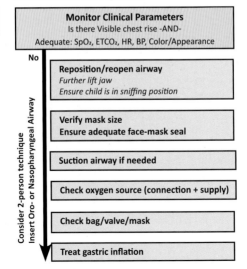

**Monitor Clinical Parameters**
Is there Visible chest rise -AND-
Adequate: SpO₂, ETCO₂, HR, BP, Color/Appearance

No

Consider 2-person technique
Insert Oro- or Nasopharyngeal Airway

**Reposition/reopen airway**
*Further lift jaw*
*Ensure child is in sniffing position*

**Verify mask size**
**Ensure adequate face-mask seal**

**Suction airway if needed**

**Check oxygen source (connection + supply)**

**Check bag/valve/mask**

**Treat gastric inflation**

## ■ Airway Adjuncts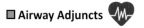

### Oropharyngeal Airway (OPA, Oral Airway)
- Indicated to relieve upper airway obstruction.  DO NOT use in patients who are conscious or semi-conscious.
- **Choosing a correct size is critical:  the tip of the OPA should extend from the corner of the mouth to the angle of the jaw**
- Too large may block the airway and/or cause trauma
- Too small may push the tongue into the oropharynx, creating an obstruction
- Insertion: Gently insert the OPA (some clinicians insert the OPA upside down, then gently rotate to fit into place)

### Nasopharyngeal Airway (NPA, Nasal Airway)
- Indicated to relieve upper airway obstruction.
- **Choosing a correct size is critical:  measure from earlobe to the tip of the nostril**
- Too large may block the airway and/or cause trauma
- Too small may not adequately relieve the obstruction
- Insertion: Gently twist while inserting the NPA into either nare, taking extreme care passing through the turbinates, until flange is flush against nare
- If leaving in place monitor skin integrity closely, and rotate between nares regularly

> **See Oakes' Respiratory Care Pocket Guide:**
> - Active cycle of breathing
> - Airway and chest oscillatory devices
> - Autogenic drainage
> - Breathing exercises
> - Incentive spirometry
> - Intermittent positive pressure breathing (IPPB)
> - Therapeutic coughing techniques

Pediatric

Procedures

## ■ Suctioning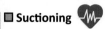

### Airway Suctioning

- Suction recommendations vary. PALS recommends a maximum of -80 to -120 mm Hg for suctioning of the airways. Other sources recommend -80 to -100 mm Hg for pediatric patients.
- Give oxygen pre- and post-suctioning
- Limit attempts to 10 seconds unless the airway is obstructed
- Monitor HR, SpO₂, and appearance during suctioning
- If bradycardia develops or appearance deteriorates, stop suction attempt. Consider use of high flow O₂ or BVM.
- If inutubated: do not advance suction catheter beyond end of ET tube

### Hazards

- Hypoxia
- Bradycardia (from vagal stimulation)
- Gagging and vomiting
- Trauma to soft tissue

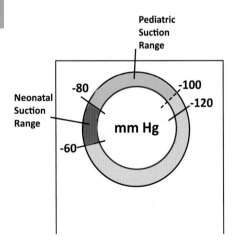

## ■ Intubation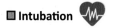

### Intubation Procedure

Prepare equipment and assess patient:

- Monitoring equipment (EKG, SpO₂, BP)
- EtCO₂ detector (or capnography)
- IV and/or IO equipment
- Bag Valve Mask (and oxygen supply)
- Suction equipment
- Oral and Nasopharyngeal airways
- Endotracheal tubes

| Age Range | Uncuffed (ID mm) | Cuffed (ID mm) |
|-----------|------------------|----------------|
| < 1 years | 3.5 | 3.0 |
| 1-2 years | 4.0 | 3.5 |
| > 2 years | 4 + (age/4) | 3.5 + (age/4) |

- Cuffed or uncuffed is acceptable in most cases
- With ↓ CL, ↑ Raw, large glottic air leak, a cuffed tube may be preferred
- Minimum of expected size, plus 1 size smaller, 1 size larger
- Laryngoscope (Miller, Macintosh) - or video laryngoscope
- Cuff pressure monitor
- 3 mL, 5 mL, 10 mL syringes
- Tube holder or tape

### Considerations

- Have all possible equipment at bedside to anticipate difficulties (fiberoptic equipment, bronchoscope, etc.)
- Cautious Rapid Sequence Intubation (RSI) in pts who are obese, who are known difficult intubations, etc.
- Pulse Oximetry, Blood Pressure, and EKG must be monitored during intubation. Interrupt attempt if oxygenation/ventilation is needed
- Only direct visualization is completely reliable. Use all possible verification methods. IF IN DOUBT, PULL IT OUT
- Remove tube at once if gurgling in stomach, and no chest expansion

## Successful Intubation Checklist:

|  | Lungs: Adequate and equal chest rise<br>Bilateral breath sounds |
|---|---|
|  | Abdomen: ↓ sounds in abdomen; no ↑ distention |
|  | Exhaled $CO_2$ (ETCO₂)—Esophageal detector device if ETCO2 not available (children > 20 kg and perfusing) |
|  | SpO₂ adequate[1] |
|  | Visualize ET Tube with laryngoscope if doubts |
|  | Chest X-Ray |

[1] It may take up to 3 minutes for SpO₂ to drop—this is not a definitive way of ensuring tube placement. SpO₂ also assumes good perfusion.

### student tip

### DOPE mnemonic
*Sudden Deterioration of Intubated Patient*

| **D**isplacement of tube | Extubated (above vocal cords)<br>Advanced (mainstem bronchi) |
|---|---|
| **O**bstruction of tube | • Secretions, blood, pus<br>• Foreign body/object<br>• Kinking of ET tube |
| **P**neumothorax | <u>Simple</u>: sudden ↓ SpO₂, ↓ chest expansion and breath sounds on affected side<br><br><u>Tension</u>: Above + hypotension, ↓ CO<br>Tracheal shift away |
| **E**quipment Failure | Multiple possible causes:<br>• O₂ supply disconnected<br>• Leak in ventilator circuit<br>• Ventilator failure (power supply, etc.)<br>• Valve malfunction (bag, vent) |

• Consider manually ventilating patient while assessing DOPE
• Some clinicians add an S to DOPE for asthmatic patients (S stands for *Stacked Breaths*)

# ◻ Tracheostomy

## Indications
- To facilitate prolonged mechanical ventilation
- To bypass an airway obstruction
- To facilitate ongoing pulmonary hygiene needs (in infants/children unable to manage sufficiently independently)

## Pediatric Tracheostomy Tubes
Tracheostomy tubes vary in design by manufacturer and purpose. Pediatric and neonatal tubes use the same sizing guide (roughly equivalent to inner diameter), but pediatric tubes are longer. Tubes also vary by:
- Material (rigid versus soft)
- Angle (arched versus angled)
- Cuff (cuffed [foam, low-pressure, tight-to-shaft] versus uncuffed)

## Tracheostomy Tube Changes
Trach changes are routine in children. It is always advisable to have 2 people at the bedside for a trach change. Take time to position the patient into an optimal position (neck slightly hyperextended).
- BVM with appropriately-sized mask
- Tracheostomy tube (and obturator): correct size + 1 size smaller
- Trach tie
- 2x2 gauze (for placement under trach)

**Average Pediatric Tracheostomy Tube Sizes**

| Weight or Age Range | Inner Diameter (mm) |
|---------------------|---------------------|
| < 1000 g | 2.5 mm |
| 1000-2500 g | 3 mm |
| 0-6 months | 3-3.5 mm |
| 6 months - 1 year | 3.5-4 mm |
| 1-2 years | 4-4.5 |
| > 2 years | (age[years] + 16) / 4 |

# Tracheostomy Troubleshooting

**Change in Clinical Status**

Δ in phonation ability

Δ in vital signs
(↓ SpO2, ↑ or ↓ HR)

Noted respiratory distress

Inability to ventilate/suction

Δ in ventilator parameters
(↑ PIP, ↓ Vt)

| Complication | Possible Causes | Possible Actions |
|---|---|---|
| Bleeding | TI Fistula (life-threatening)<br>Suction trauma<br>Tracheitis<br>Granulation | Consult MD |
| Chest pain | Cardiac<br>Misplaced trach<br>Occluded trach<br>Respiratory failure | Request EKG<br>Verify trach placement |
| Crackling/Edema around stoma | Misplaced trach (in tissue) | Verify placement<br>Change trach |
| Difficulty passing suction catheter | Catheter too large<br>Misplaced trach<br>Occluded trach | Consider lavaging<br>If still unable to pass suction and/or patient distress, immediately decannulate |
| Excessive coughing and gagging | Excessive secretions<br>Tolerance of trach | Bronchial hygiene<br>Check trach tie<br>Place on ventilator |

# ■ Airway Clearance

There are many airway clearance adjuncts approved for use (inlcuding Flutter valves, Acapella device, etc.). This content is covered in-depth in Oakes' Respiratory Care Pocket Guide (RespiratoryBooks.com).

# Chest Physiotherapy (CPT)

| Postural Drainage (See Diagrams following pages) | |
|---|---|
| **Indications** | Particularly beneficial in Cystic Fibrosis, May benefit patients with thick, secretions (?) |
| **Technique** | • Perform at least 1 hr before or 2 hrs after meals.<br>• Prescribed bronchodilator therapy should be given 15 min before therapy.<br>• Ensure patient loosens any tight or binding clothing.<br>• Drainage should begin with superior segments and progress downward. Lung segment to be drained should be placed such that main bronchus is pointing ↓ (use of pillows/blankets may assist in positioning)<br>• Maintain position for 3-20 min, depending on quantity and tenacity of secretions and patient tolerance. Limit total treatment time to 30-40 min.<br>• Appply Percussion and Vibration (see next page)<br>• Have patient cough q 5 min during each position and after therapy (use FET in head down positions). There will be less of a rise in ICP if pt is in upright position during cough. |
| **Monitoring** | • Watch for signs of patient intolerance and monitor heart rate, BP, and $SpO_2$ during treatment<br>• Signs of respiratory compromise:<br>    • ↓ diaphragm excusion in head-down position<br>    • Airway obstruction from secretions/collapse<br>• ALL THERAPY SHOULD BE ADJUSTED BASED UPON PATIENT'S CLINICAL CONDITION / TOLERANCE |
| **Clinical Notes** | • Oxygen requirements may increase during CPT, but should decrease following. Positional changes will alter V/Q and may be either beneficial or detrimental to Oxygenation/Ventilation<br>• **NOTE**: Owing to the potential detrimental side effects and recent evidence showing a beneficial effect of using modified positioning, head-down positioning is no longer recommended to be used with PD&P in neo/peds by the CF Foundation and various guidelines in Australia, Canada, and Europe. |

| Percussion and Vibration | |
| --- | --- |
| **Indications** | Particularly beneficial in Cystic Fibrosis; may benefit patients with thick, secretions |
| **Technique** | • Percussion is applied to various lung segments either manually (with cupped hands) or mechanically with a motorized percussor/vibrator type unit (electric or pneumatic).<br>• Chest percussion or clapping and vibration are often used in conjunction with postural drainage.<br>• Percussion or clapping is usually applied for several minutes or as tolerated by the patient.<br>• The therapist should remove any jewelry that might interfere with percussion technique.<br>• Vibration is applied to the chest area with hands tensing at 6-8 vibrations per second for 4-6 exhalations.<br>• The procedure concludes with a deep cough (several techniques are described in this chapter) and expulsion of secretions.<br>• Patients should be allowed to rest as each lung segment is drained and cleared.<br>• Should not be performed on a bare chest, over heart, stomach, spine, kidneys, adolescents' breasts, chest tubes, incisions, wounds, fractures. |

Pediatric

Procedures

# External Anatomy of Lungs

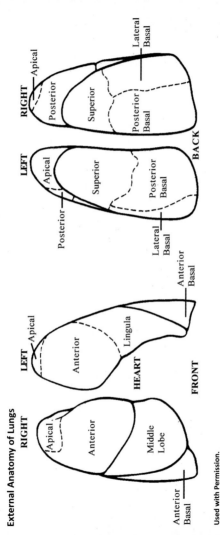

**RIGHT**

Apical

Anterior

Middle Lobe

Anterior Basal

**LEFT**

Apical

Anterior

Lingula

**HEART**

**FRONT**

Anterior Basal

**LEFT**

Apical

Posterior

Superior

Posterior Basal

Lateral Basal

**RIGHT**

Apical

Posterior

Superior

Posterior Basal

Lateral Basal

**BACK**

**Used with Permission.**
An introduction to postural drainage and percussion. In (2012). Cystic Fibrosis Foundation.

## Postural Drainage Modified Positions (Cystic Fibrosis Foundation)

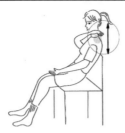

### Upper Lobes (Self Percussion)

Patient should sit upright. Instruct pt to percuss area between collarbone and top of shoulder blade, being careful to avoid bony structures.

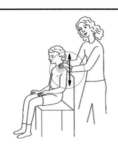

### Upper Front Chest

Patient should sit upright. Percuss area between collarbone and top of shoulderblade, being careful to avoid bony structures.

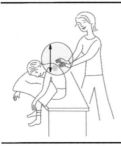

### Upper Back Chest

Pt should sit upright, leaning forward at about 30 degrees. Stand behind pt and percuss both sides of upper back, being careful to avoid bony structures.

**Used with Permission. Text adapted.**

An Introduction to Postural Drainage & Percussion (2012). Cystic Fibrosis Foundation. More information can be found at www.cff.org.

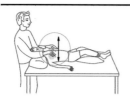

### Upper Front Chest

Patient should be supine, with arms to sides. Percuss bilaterally between collar-bone and nipple line.

Avoid bony structures and breasts on females.

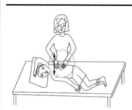

### Left Side Front Chest

Patient should be on right side, with left arm over head if able. Percuss over lower ribs, just below nipple line on front of chest.

Avoid abdomen and breasts on females.

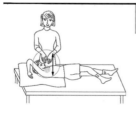

### Right Side Front Chest

Patient should be on left side, with right arm over head if able. Percuss over lower ribs, just below nipple line on front of chest.

Avoid abdomen and breasts on females

**Used with Permission. Text adapted.**

An introduction to postural drainage and percussion. In (2012). Cystic Fibrosis Foundation.

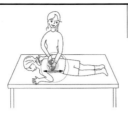

### Lower Back Chest

Patient should be proned. Percuss bilaterally at bottom of chest wall (use bottom edge of ribcage as a guide)

Avoid bony stuctures (lower ribcage and vertebral column)

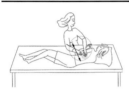

### Left Lower Side Back Chest

Pt should be positioned on right side, rolled forward 1/4 turn. Percuss lower left side of chest above bottom edge or ribs

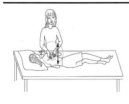

### Right Lower Side Back

Patient should be positioned on left side, rolled forward 1/4 turn. Percuss lower right side of chest above bottom edge of ribs

**Used with Permission. Text adapted.**

An introduction to postural drainage and percussion. In (2012). Cystic Fibrosis Foundation.

Pediatric

Procedures

## Traditional Postural Drainage Positions

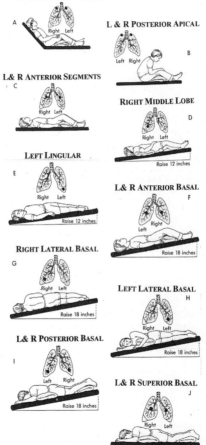

L & R ANTERIOR APICAL

A

Right  Left

L & R POSTERIOR APICAL

B

Left  Right

L & R ANTERIOR SEGMENTS

C

Right  Left

RIGHT MIDDLE LOBE

D

Right  Left

Raise 12 inches

LEFT LINGULAR

E

Right  Left

Raise 12 inches

L & R ANTERIOR BASAL

F

Left  Right

Raise 18 inches

RIGHT LATERAL BASAL

G

Right  Left

Raise 18 inches

LEFT LATERAL BASAL

H

Right  Left

Raise 18 inches

L & R POSTERIOR BASAL

I

Left  Right

Raise 18 inches

L & R SUPERIOR BASAL

J

Right  Left

Adapted from Hirsch, J. and Hannock, L. *Mosby's Manual of Clinical Nursing Practice.* Copyright 1985 by Mosby.

| In-Exsufflator (Cof-flator™ or Cough Assist™ ) | |
|---|---|
| **Description** | Applies a positive pressure to the airway (mask or tube) and then rapidly shifts to a negative pressure producing a high expiratory flow rate from the lungs stimulating a cough. |
| **Indications** | The inability to effectively cough or clear secretions as a result of reduced peak expiratory flow rates (< 5-6 L/s) as seen in high spinal cord injuries, neuro-muscular conditions, or fatigue associated with intrinsic lung disorders. |
| **Contra-indications** | • Recent barotrauma, or patients prone to pneumothorax or pneumomediastinum.<br>• Patients with cardiovascular instability should be monitored with $SpO_2$ and heart rate. |
| **Directions for use** | • Patients are usually given 4-5 coughing cycles in succession, followed by a 30 second rest period.<br>• There are usually 6-10 cycles for a full treatment.<br>• A typical cycle consists of the following:<br>  • The unit slowly builds up positive pressure in the chest over a 1-3 sec period to about + 40 mm Hg.<br>  • It then rapidly switches to the "exhale" mode with a drop in pressure to -40 mm Hg in 0.02 seconds (total drop of 80 mm Hg).<br>  • Exhalation pressure is usually held for 2-3 sec.<br>  • This results in a cough and expectoration of secretions.<br>• The device can be titrated to maximum insufflation by chest wall excursion, auscultaion, and patient comfort.<br>• Some models allow for "Manual" versus "Automatic" modes. In automatic mode, inspiratory and expiratory times and pressures are set as well as a pause in between breaths. In manual mode, pressures are set, while timing is via switching from Inspiration to expiration - breathing at the same rate with the patient can be helpful in synchronizing.<br>• May be used by mouthpiece or mask, as well as by tracheostomy. |

Pediatric

Procedures

| Positive Expiratory Pressure (PEP) Therapy | |
|---|---|
| Description | Positive expiratory pressure (PEP therapy) is the active exhalation against a variable flow resistor reaching pressures of ~ 10-20 cm $H_2O$. |
| Indications | PEP Therapy enhances bronchial hygiene therapy by improving airway patency and airflow through airways that are partially obstructed by stenting the airways and/or increasing intrathoracic pressure distal to retained secretions, which:<br>• Reduces air-trapping in susceptible patients<br>• Promotes increased mobilization and clearance of secretions from the airways<br>• Enhances collateral ventilation and opens airways behind mucus obstructions, improving pulm. mech. & facilitating gas exchange<br>Secondarily, it may help prevent or reverse atelectasis, prevent recurrent infection, and slow disease progression. |
| Devices | Often a disposable, single-patient use device that is self-administered. It is less time-consuming and does not require the precise positioning of chest physical therapy. Used with FET ("huff coughing"). |
| Procedure | 1. Instruct to sit upright, with a tight seal around mouthpiece/mask, then inhale, using the diaphragm, to a volume > VT (but not TLC).<br>2. Instruct to exhale actively, but not forcefully, to FRC, achieving an airway pressure of 10-20 cm $H_2O$*. I:E ratio 1:3, 1:4<br>3. Perform 10-20 breaths through the device, then 2-5 huff coughs.<br>4. Repeat cycle 5-10 times (15-20 minutes) or until secretions are cleared.<br><br>*The amount of PEP varies with the size of the adjustable orifice and the level of expiratory flow generated by the patient. Adjust to meet patient's need. |
| Oscillatory PEP | The combination of PEP therapy with airway vibrations or oscillations. See following pages. |

| Acapella™ | |
|---|---|
| **Description** | A disposable, single-patient use device (self-administered) that delivers positive expiratory pressure with high frequency oscillations<br><br>*Vibratory Positive Expiratory Pressure Therapy* |
| **Directions** | Patient exhales air through an opening that is periodically closed by a pivoting cone. As air passes through the opening, the cone will open and close the airflow path. This produces a vibratory pressure waveform - allowing secretions to be mobilized and expectorated. |
| **Settings** | Dial on end of device sets vibration/oscillation frequency (6-20 Hz). Device is available in three flow rate ranges |

| Flutter Device™ | |
|---|---|
| **Description** | A device which produces oscillations in expiratory pressure and airflow. The resultant vibration of the airways loosens mucus from the airway walls. |
| **Contra-indications** | Patients with pneumothorax or right heart failure |
| **Directions** | • Patient seated with back straight, head tilted slightly back or seated with elbows resting on a table with head tilted slightly back<br>• Initially, stem is positioned horizontally. Then adjusted up or down to get the maximum "fluttering" effect within the patient's chest (Vibrations can be felt by placing one hand on back and the other on the front of chest)<br>• Patient takes a deep breath (but not to TLC), holds for 2-3 seconds, then exhales actively (but not forcefully) as long as possible while keeping cheeks as hard and flat as possible<br>• Exhale repeatedly through the device until coughing is stimulated.<br>• Continue for approximately 15 minutes or until patient feels no additional mucus can be raised<br>• Perform procedure 2-4 times/day or as directed |

| Intrapulmonary Percussive Ventilation™ (IPV) | |
|---|---|
| **Description** | The delivery of high-frequency percussive breaths (sub-tidal volume) into the patient's airways by a pneumatic device |
| **Indications** | The inability to effectively cough or clear secretions as a result of reduced peak expiratory flow rates |
| **Contra-indications** | Bronchospasm, lung contusion, pneumothorax, pulmonary hemorrhage, subcutaneous emphysema, TB, vomiting and aspiration |
| **Directions** | • Patient breathes through a mouthpiece or artificial airway and the unit delivers high flow rate bursts of gas into the lungs from 100-300 x/min. Continuous positive pressure is maintained (typically 15-40 cm H2O) while the pulses dilate the airways. At the end of the percussive inspiratory cycle (5-10 sec), a deep exhalation is performed with expectoration of secretions.<br>• Normal treatment time is 20 min. Aerosols (bland or medicated) may also be delivered via the attached nebulizer with this therapy. |
| **Settings** | • Pressure is set via a manometer with optimum range being 30-40 cmH2O (less for ↑ Compliance, more for ↓ Compliance). This is equivalent to setting a "Mean Airway Pressure."<br>• Difficulty knob changes the frequency of the oscillations, which may improve clearance and recruitment. It is recommended that this knob be turned back and forth every few minutes during treatment. |
| **Notes** | • This therapy can be done as an adjunct to mechanical ventilation (in-line with ventilator circuit)<br>• When effective, several breaks may need to be taken in order to get pt to cough or suction<br>• Many clinicians recommend utilizing an inline suction catheter when used in conjunction with an artificial airway to facilitate suctioning<br>• Cuffed artificial airways: Suction above cuff, and then at least partially deflate cuff during tx to facilitate secretion clearance |

| Vest Airway Clearance System™ | |
|---|---|
| Description | • The system includes an air pulse generator, inflatable vest, and connecting tube<br>• It provides high frequency chest wall compressions which help mobilize secretion |
| Indications | • Follow the guidelines established by the AARC for airway clearance therapies.<br>• A patient-specific assessment should always be used weighing potential benefits and risks.<br>• Indications include cystic fibrosis, bronchiectasis, or conditions where the patient has the inability to effectively mobilize and expectorate secretions. |
| Contra-indications | Active hemorrhage, cardiac instability, chest wall pain, lung contusion, recent thoracic skin grafts, recently placed pacemaker, subcutaneous emphysema, suspectedtuberculosis, unstabilized head and/or neck injury. |
| Directions | • As the patient wears the inflatable vest, small gas volumes alternately flow into and out of the unit – rapidly inflating and deflating (compressing and releasing) the chest wall to create air flow and cough- like shear forces to move secretions<br>• Timing of the pulse is manually controlled by the patient or clinician<br>• The intensity (25-40 mm Hg) and frequency (5-25 Hz) of the pulses can also be adjusted by the patient or clinician |
| Notes | • The vest is often used with chronic lung conditions, including cystic fibrosis. Working with the patient to ensure an appropriate/comfortable fit, and developing plans for integrating into their life routine, is critical in establishing compliance. |

## Airway Clearance
## Selection Algorithm

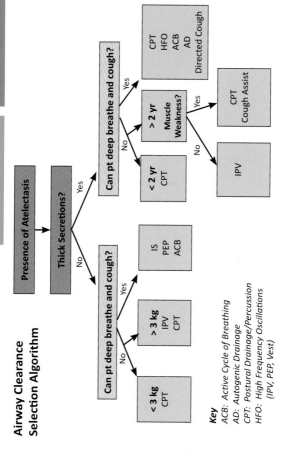

**Key**
ACB: *Active Cycle of Breathing*
AD: *Autogenic Drainage*
CPT: *Postural Drainage/Percussion*
HFO: *High Frequency Oscillations*
      *(IPV, PEP, Vest)*

## ■ Oxygen Delivery Devices

| Delivery System | Liter flow[1] | O2 % delivered | Comments | Cautions |
|---|---|---|---|---|
| **Low Flow System** (Delivers 100% O2 at flows < patient's inspiratory (demand). Room air is entrained, total patient demand is not met, and FIO2 is highly variable.) | | | | |
| Nasal Cannula | 1-6 L/min | 24-40% | Delivers approximately 4%/L, comfortable, good for low %, inexpensive, patient can eat, talk, and sleep. | ↓ FIO2: as $\dot{V}_E$↑, need patent nasal passages, use humidifier ≥ 4 L/min, easily dislodged, may cause irritation, dryness, or nosebleed. |
| Nasal Catheter | 1-6 L/min | 24-45% | Same as cannula | Same as cannula, plus must be changed every 8 hours, clogs easily, abdominal distention. |
| Simple Mask | 5-10 L/min | 35-50% | Delivers approx. 4%/L, FIO2 variable depending on fit and ventilation variables., hot/uncomfortable, interferes with eating/talking. | Need minimum 5 L/min to flush $CO_2$ from mask, more skin irritation |
| Partial Rebreathing Mask | 6-10 L/min | 40-70% | High % delivered, same as simple mask, FIO2 variable depending on fit | $\dot{V}$ should be set to keep reservoir > 1/3 – 1/2 full upon inspiration. |

| Delivery System | Liter flow[1] | O₂% delivered | Comments | Cautions |
|---|---|---|---|---|
| **Non-Rebreathing Mask** | ≥ 10 L/min | 60-80% | Same as partial rebreathing mask | Same as partial rebreathing mask |
| **High Flow System** (High air flow with oxygen enrichment [HAFOE] which may meet the total demand of the patient [should be ≥ 60 L/min]) | | | | |
| **Air Entrainment Mask (Venturi)** | Variable | 24-50% | Exact O₂ concentrations, can be adapted to deliver aerosol, device of choice for patients on O₂ drive. | Entrainment ports easily occluded. |

### AIR ENTRAINMENT RATIOS

| O₂% | Air/O₂ ratio |     | O₂% | Air/O₂ ratio |
|---|---|---|---|---|
| 24% | 25/1 | | 50% | 1.7/1 |
| 28% | 10/1 | | 60% | 1/1 |
| 30% | 8/1 | | 70% | 0.6/1 |
| 35% | 5/1 | | 80% | 0.3/1 |
| 40% | 3/1 | | | |

**Calculating Oxygen Blending Ratios & Entrainment Ratios – See Oakes' Respiratory Care Pocket Guide**

| Delivery System | Liter flow[1] | O₂% delivered | Comments | Cautions |
|---|---|---|---|---|
| **Air Entrainment Nebulizer** or **High-Volume Humidifier** | 8-40 L/min | 28-100% | Used to deliver precise O₂ and/ or aerosol, high O₂%, can provide controlled temperature of gas. FIO₂ determined by the nebulization system and flow rate or blender. | Use with aerosol mask, face tent, T-piece, trach mask or collar. May need two or three setups to meet inspiratory flow when FIO₂ > 50% Hazards of aerosol: condensation in tubing |

| Delivery System | Liter flow[1] | O₂% delivered | Comments | Cautions |
|---|---|---|---|---|
| High-flow Therapy Systems | Neonatal: 1- 8 L/min<br><br>Pediatric: 8-20 L/min<br><br>Adolescent: 20-60 L/min | 21% - 100% | Used to deliver precise O₂ and humidification from 80% to 100% RH at body temp (37° C).<br>FIO₂ is determined by analysis via bleed-in or blender.<br><br>Beneficial in pulmonary fibrosis, CHF, asthma, cystic fibrosis and post-surgical care where low-flow oxygen or other delivery systems is inadequate<br><br>Can also be used in humidifying CPAP, improving pulmonary hygiene, tracheostomy management and in the treatment of rhinitis/sinusitis. | Use with a special large-bore nasal cannula to accommodate high liter flows.<br><br>Recommended for neo/ped pts with oxygenation difficulties related to BPD, CF and other pulm conditions w/ PaO₂ < 55 mmHg or SpO2 < 88%, tachypnea, retractions, mild apnea and/or bradycardia (AOP).<br><br>Use in conjunction with SpO₂ monitoring<br><br>May create variable CPAP effect<br>(some estimate as much as 1 cmH20 per 10 L/min, though may vary widely by device, physiology, etc.) |

| Heliox Therapy (Helium - Oxygen) | |
|---|---|
| Function | Helium reduces the resistance of air/O₂ flowing through narrowed airways. Its primary value is in the tx of airway obstruction by enhancing the delivery of O₂ and aerosol to the distal areas of the lung.<br>Helium can be used as a temporizing agent to reduce WOB and allow time for the more standard forms of therapy to reach peak effect. |
| Indications | • Acute exacerbations of asthma<br>• Post extubation stridor<br>• Status asthmaticus<br>• Tracheal stenosis/Upper airway obstruction |
| Benefits | • Improved homogeneity of gas distribution resulting in:<br>   • ↑ alveolar ventilation, oxygenation and V$_T$<br>   • ↓ WOB, PaCO₂, gas trapping, auto-PEEP, PIP and Pplat, barotrauma, I:E ratios, and shunting<br>• Movement of the equal-pressure point of the airways upstream |
| Common Mixtures | • 80% He / 20% O₂<br>• 70% He / 30% O₂ *<br>(* Used when O₂ therapy is indicated for hypoxemia. If FIO₂ > 0.6 is required, He/O₂ will have little effect) |
| Admin-istration | **Spontaneous breathing**: Deliver via tight-fit NRB. May add O₂ nasal cannula to titrate to desired SpO₂.<br><br>**Intubated**: Deliver as adjunct via ventilator<br><br>**Delivery using an O₂ flowmeter requires flow conversion:**<br>   70/30:  set flow x 1.6 = total flow delivered<br>   80/20:  set flow x 1.8 = total flow delivered |

| Monitoring | ABG sampling<br>Arrhythmia<br>Dyspnea (WOB & SOB) | Heart rate<br>Pulse oximetry<br>Pulsus paradoxus |
|---|---|---|
| Hazards | Anoxia- analyze delivered gas<br>Barotrauma- via non-heliox ventilators | Too ↑ or too ↓ bronchodilator - too ↓ or ↑ of a flow through the neb<br>Hypothermia - via hood on infants |

| Hypoxic Gas Delivery (Mixtures) | |
|---|---|
| **Function** | Delivery of $FIO_2$ < 0.21 (21%) with the goal of causing hypoxic vasoconstriction, which leads to a decrease in pulmonary vascular resistance. |
| **Indications** | Single-ventricle cardiac defects, including hypoplastic left-heart syndrome |
| **Admin-istration** | Gas is blended externally and then delivered via mechanical ventilation or oxygen hood. Ventilator: Air hose is usually connected to a Nitrogen tank (with 50 PSI outlet) |
| **Monitoring** | Close monitoring and careful setting of $O_2$ alarm (usually utilizing an external oxygen analyzer) is important |
| **Hazards** | Cerebral effects are possbie Usually requires overriding built-in ventilator safety systems |

## ☐ Inhaled Nitric Oxide (pediatric considerations)
### See section starting on page 5-18 for detailed information

**Inhaled Nitric Oxide (iNO)**

iNO may be indicated in PICU patients who are in Acute Hypoxemic Respiratory Failure (measured by an Arterial Blood Gas with Oxygen Index > 15 or P/F Ratio ≤ 100)

### Inhaled Nitric Oxide Pediatric Management Algorithm

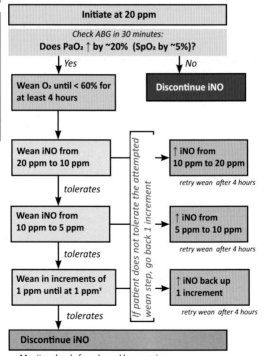

Monitor closely for rebound hypoxemia -
Consider ↑ $O_2$% by 10% prior to discontinuation

| Nitrous Oxide | |
|---|---|
| Function | Used in procedural sedation, results in amnesia and mild-to-moderate analgesia. |
| Benefits | Onset of action is short (< 1 minute) <br> Recovery is fast (< 20 minutes) |
| Admin-istration | 1:1 mixture of oxygen and nitrous oxide are administered via a handheld mask |
| Monitoring | Close monitoring is indicated.  While respiratory deterioration is unlikely, it is important to have appropriate airway management equipment available (see procedural sedation section) |
| Hazards | Use with caution in patients with obstructive lung disease |

# ☐ Procedural Sedation (Conscious)

*The process of administering a sedative to depress the level of consciousness with the goal of not depressing the drive to breathe or affecting airway patency. There is a fine line that exists between the elements.*

**Key Concepts:**
- Goal is to create comfort and gain cooperation
- Levels: Minimum, Moderate, Deep
- Many factors affect pain and pain perception in children (age, developmental age, previous experiences, bedside rapport, etc.)
  - Often children < 6-years-old and those with developmental disabilities require deeper levels of sedation
  - Older children may require less deep levels of sedation with parental presence, distraction, topical local anesthetics, and guided imagery exercises
- Response to analgesia is individual. This further emphasizes the importance of close monitoring and being prepared for respiratory depression.
- Drug absorption, distribution, and elimination vary greatly with age (primarily due to ↑ lipids as a child ages), as well as changes in renal and hepatic elimination
- Analgesics and sedatives are usually given at the lowest dose in the therapeutic range and then titrated up for efffect

## Indications

### Diagnostics
- Lumbar Puncture (LP)
- Arthrocentesis
- Bone marrow biopsy
- Sexual assault examination
- Imaging: CT or MRI
- Multiple procedures required (IV, catheter placement, etc.)

### Therapeutics
- Foreign body removal
- Dislocations and reductions
- Debridements
- Suturing

## Pre-Procedure

- Develop rapport with the child and caretaker(s)
- Assess the patient
- Inspect airway (see Mallampati scoring, page 12-5)
- Collect relevant medical history (including allergies)

## "SOAPME" Preparation Checklist[1]

Key equipment (in red) should be set-up.
All other equipment should be available, but not set-up.

| | |
|---|---|
| **S** | **Suction:**<br>• Oral suction<br>• Suction catheters (appropriate sizes)<br>• Suction source |
| **O** | **Oxygen delivery equipment:**<br>• Bag-Valve-Mask connected to oxygen flowmeter<br>• Nasal cannula<br>• Nonrebreather mask<br>• Oxygen source (flowmeter, wall outlet or cylinder) |
| **A** | **Airways:**<br>• Naso- and oropharyngeal airway (various sizes)<br>• Intubation equipment<br>• Laryngoscope (and blades)—verify function<br>• Endotracheal tubes (various sizes)<br>• Difficult intubation equipment should be easily assessible if needed |
| **P** | **Pharmacy:**<br>• PALS drugs (or code cart)<br>• Reversal agents (when appropriate) |
| **M** | **Monitoring:**<br>• SpO$_2$, EKG, NIBP, ETCO$_2$, auscultation |
| **E** | **Equipment:**<br>• Defibrillator with appropriate size pads<br>• Other specialized equipment/drugs specific to needs of this patient |

[1] Summarized and adapted from American Academy of Pediatrics Guidelines

**Procedural Sedation Intervention Algorithm**

**Detect Hypoventilation Early**
↑ ETCO$_2$, ↓ SpO$_2$, ↓ RR, ↓ HR, ↓ Chest Rise

Instruct to deep breathe

Position patient (sniffing)

Perform jaw thrust

Suction (as indicated)

Place nasal airway

Positive Pressure Ventilation

Place oral airway

Intubate

continued deterioration

Stop Drugs, ↑ O$_2$

Consider reversal agents

| Symptomatic Bradycardia | Give atropine |
| Hypotension | Give IV fluids |
| Hemodynamic Instability | PALS/Call code |

- Not all steps will necessarily be performed in order
- Most deterioration is reversed by focusing on patient position, jaw thrust, and competent bag-valve-mask technique

# Index

# Find all of our titles

## Buy direct from the publisher: low pricing and the latest editions

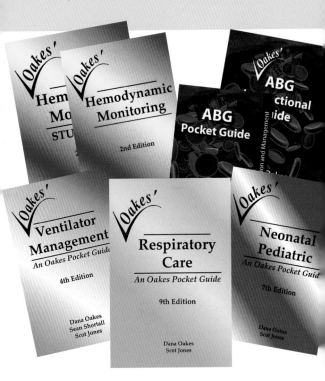

**RespiratoryBooks.com**